ALTERNATIVE MEDICINE AND WELLNESS TECHNIQUES

Scholarly Articles by Peter Fritz Walter

The Law of Evidence

The Restriction of National Sovereignty

Alternative Medicine and Wellness Techniques

Consciousness and Shamanism

Creative Prayer

Soul Jazz

The Ego Matter

The Star Script

The Lunar Bull

Basics of Mythology

Basics of Feng Shui

Power or Depression?

The Mythology of Narcissism

Normative Psychoanalysis

Notes on Consciousness

Patterns of Perception

Sane Child vs. Insane Society

Basics of the Science of Mind

The Secret Science

Oedipal Hero

Processed Reality

ALTERNATIVE MEDICINE AND WELLNESS TECHNIQUES

14 Paths to Integral Health

by Peter Fritz Walter

Published by Sirius-C Media Galaxy LLC

113 Barksdale Professional Center, Newark, Delaware, USA

©2015 Peter Fritz Walter. Some rights reserved.

2017 Revised, Updated and Reformatted Edition.

Creative Commons Attribution 4.0 International License

This publication may be distributed, used for an adaptation or for derivative works, also for commercial purposes, as long as the rights of the author are attributed. The attribution must be given to the best of the user's ability with the information available. Third party licenses or copyright of quoted resources are untouched by this license and remain under their own license.

The moral right of the author has been asserted

Set in Palatino

Designed by Peter Fritz Walter

ISBN 978-1-515235-24-8

Publishing Categories
Medical / Alternative Medicine

Publisher Contact Information
publisher@sirius-c-publishing.com
http://sirius-c-publishing.com

Author Contact Information
pfw@peterfritzwalter.com

About Dr. Peter Fritz Walter
http://peterfritzwalter.com

About the Author

Parallel to an international law career in Germany, Switzerland and the United States, Dr. Peter Fritz Walter (Pierre) focused upon fine art, cookery, astrology, musical performance, social sciences and humanities.

He started writing essays as an adolescent and received a high school award for creative writing and editorial work for the school magazine.

After finalizing his law diplomas, he graduated with an LL.M. in European Integration at Saarland University, Germany, in 1982, and with a Doctor of Law title from University of Geneva, Switzerland, in 1987.

He then took courses in psychology at the University of Geneva and interviewed a number of psychotherapists in Lausanne and Geneva, Switzerland. His interest was intensified through a hypnotherapy with an Ericksonian American hypnotherapist in Lausanne. This led him to the recovery and healing of his inner child.

After a second career as a corporate trainer and personal coach, Pierre retired in 2004 as a full-time writer, philosopher and consultant.

His nonfiction books emphasize a systemic, holistic, cross-cultural and interdisciplinary perspective, while his fiction works and short stories focus upon education, philosophy, perennial wisdom, and the poetic formulation of an integrative worldview.

Pierre is a German-French bilingual native speaker and writes English as his 4th language after German, Latin and French. He also reads source literature for his research works in Spanish, Italian, Portuguese, and Dutch. In addition, Pierre has notions of Thai, Khmer, Chinese, Japanese, and Vietnamese.

All of Pierre's books are hand-crafted and self-published, designed by the author. Pierre publishes via his Delaware company, Sirius-C Media Galaxy LLC, and under the imprints of IPUBLICA and SCM (Sirius-C Media).

*Dedicated to Paracelsus,
the earliest and greatest of all
natural healers.*

The author's profits from this book are being donated to charity.

Contents

Overview 11
The 14 Ways to Wellness

Ayurveda 12
Chinese Medicine 13
Homeopathy 13
Kirlian Photography 13
Kyudo 14
Naturopathy 14
Osteopathy 15
Qigong 15
Radionics 15
Reiki 16
Sophrology 16
Tai Chi Chuan 17
Tibetan Medicine 17
Yoga 18

Why Did I Write this Guide? 19
Personal Experiences

Ayurveda 37
The Science of Life

Traditional Chinese Medicine 43
Another Life Science

Homeopathy 61

From Paracelsus to Masaru Emoto

INTRODUCTION	61
PARACELSUS	63
SAMUEL HAHNEMANN	71
EDWARD BACH	76
MASARU EMOTO	84

KIRLIAN PHOTOGRAPHY   93
The Final Evidence of the Luminous Energy Field

KYUDO   99
A Japanese Martial Art

WHAT IS KYUDO?	99
KYUDO IN GERMANY	100
KYUDO IN JAPAN	100

NATUROPATHY   103
An American Natural Healing System

THE SIX PRINCIPLES OF HEALING	103
NATURE'S HEALING POWER	104
IDENTIFY THE CAUSE	105
DO NO HARM	106
WHOLE PERSON TREATMENT	106
THE PHYSICIAN IS TEACHER	107
DISEASE PREVENTION	107

OSTEOPATHY   109
The Eight Principles of Osteopathic Healing

WHAT IS OSTEOPATHY?	109
THE EIGHT PRINCIPLES OF OSTEOPATHY	111

CONTENTS

QIGONG — 113
The Art of Breathing
- WHAT IS QIGONG? — 114
- THE QIGONG POSTURE — 115
- QIGONG FOR HEALING SEXUAL SADISM — 116

RADIONICS — 119
The Unknown Medical Science
- WHAT IS RADIONICS? — 119

REIKI — 127
The Usui System

SOPHROLOGY — 131
The Study of the Harmony of Consciousness
- WHAT IS SOPHROLOGY? — 131
- BENEFITS — 135

TAI CHI CHUAN — 137
The Soft Martial Art
- WHAT IS TAI CHI CHUAN? — 137
- THE MOVEMENTS — 139
- THE BENEFITS — 140
- LEARNING THE TECHNIQUE — 142
- PRACTICE REGULARLY — 142
- MEANING OF THE WORD — 144

TIBETAN MEDICINE — 151
Feeling the Pulse

YOGA 155
The Two Yoga
INDIAN YOGA 155
CHINESE-THAI YOGA 156

BIBLIOGRAPHY 159
Contextual Bibliography

PERSONAL NOTES 173

OVERVIEW

The 14 Ways to Wellness

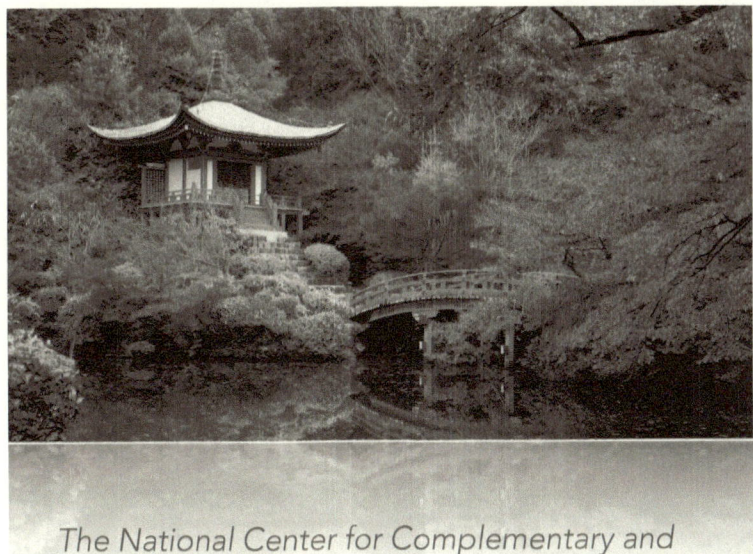

The National Center for Complementary and Alternative Medicine defines complementary and alternative medicine as a group of diverse medical and health care systems, practices, and products that are not presently considered to be part of conventional medicine. It also defines integrative medicine as combining mainstream medical therapies and CAM therapies for which there is some high-quality scientific evidence of safety and effectiveness.

As such the United States' approach to alternative medicine can be said to be well-regulated, integrative and permissive to practices that may not be part of traditional Western medicine.

The regulations in place are focused upon avoiding abusive and incompetent practices and outright charlatanism through a system of minimum requirements and professional control.

The fourteen practices I will be describing in this article are all regulated in the United States, while regulations may differ from State to State. But they are recognized as valid alternative medical practices.

Ayurveda

Ayurveda is India's oldest indigenous medical science. It is completely non-chemical and non-harmful, and highly effective. It has been promoted by Mahatma Gandhi and came to be known in the West through his writings and the British colonization of India.

OVERVIEW

Chinese Medicine

Chinese medicine and pharmacology is based on the natural flow of the *ch'i*, the bioplasmatic energy that I came to call *e-force* and that is an angular stone in the ancient Chinese system of healing illness.

Homeopathy

Homeopathy was founded by Samuel Hahnemann, and was expanded very importantly by Edward Bach.

Kirlian Photography

Kirlian Photography refers to a form of contact print photography, theoretically associated with high-voltage. It is named after the Russian physician, Dr. Semyon Kirlian, who in 1939 discovered that if an object on a photographic plate is subjected to a strong electric field, an image is created on the plate.

Kyudo

Kyudo, literally meaning way of the bow, is the Japanese art of archery. It is a modern Japanese martial art *(gendai budo)*. It is estimated that there are approximately half a million practitioners of Kyudo today.

Naturopathy

Naturopathy is a natural healing practice that is genuinely American and taught at major natural healing centers and universities in California, Arizona and Texas. While it may be taught elsewhere at reputed universities in the United States, the centers and universities in the three mentioned states are the most recognized. This has historical and climatic reasons. The plants used in naturopathy best grow in the hotter climatic regions of the North American belt.

OVERVIEW

Osteopathy

Osteopathy is equally a natural healing practice that originates from the United States.

Qigong

Qigong, or *ch'i kung*, refers to a wide variety of traditional cultivation practices that involve methods of accumulating, circulating, and working with *ch'i*, breathing or energy within the body. Qigong is practiced for health maintenance purposes, as a therapeutic intervention, as a medical profession, a spiritual path and/or component of Chinese martial arts.

Radionics

Radionics is a science that to this day is understood only by a few, as it is so far still largely located within the gray area between official science and spirituality, unknown to the great public. But that does not diminish its importance. It owns its existence to two rather distinct streams of influence, for one the esoteric spiritual teachings of Alice Bailey, on one hand, and the experimental findings of the Russian-French scientist Georges Lakhovsky, on the other.

Reiki

Reiki is a spiritual practice developed in 1922 by Mikao Usui. After three weeks of fasting and meditating on Mount Kurama, in Japan, Usui claimed to receive the ability of healing without energy depletion. A portion of the practice, *tenohira* or palm healing, is used as a form of complementary and alternative medicine (CAM). Tenohira is a technique whereby practitioners believe they are moving healing energy (a form of *ki*) through the palms.

Sophrology

Sophrology was created by Dr. Alfonso Caycedo in the 1960s. It is a branch of mindbody psychology that focuses on understanding human consciousness and altered states of consciousness for short-term or long-term positive modifications, relaxation and purposes of personal growth and creativity boosting. The term is derived from old Greek and means *study of the harmony of consciousness*.

Tai Chi Chuan

Tai Chi Chuan is an internal Chinese martial art, often promoted and practiced as a martial arts therapy for the purposes of health and longevity. Tai Chi Chuan is considered a soft style martial art, an art applied with as much deep relaxation or softness in the musculature as possible, to distinguish its theory and application from that of the hard martial art styles which use a degree of tension in the muscles.

Tibetan Medicine

Tibetan Medicine is one of the most ancient natural healing traditions in the world. Much of it is not yet known in the West. I know little about it, except that Tibetan doctors are the most trained in pulse reading and can predict diseases years ahead. So on this page I just report a personal experience.

Yoga

The Sanskrit word *Yoga* means to join or unite. It is generally translated as union of the individual atman or individual soul with paramatman or universal soul.

Yoga is a family of ancient spiritual practices dating back more than 5000 years from India. It is one of the six schools of Hindu philosophy.

Why Did I Write this Guide?

Personal Experiences

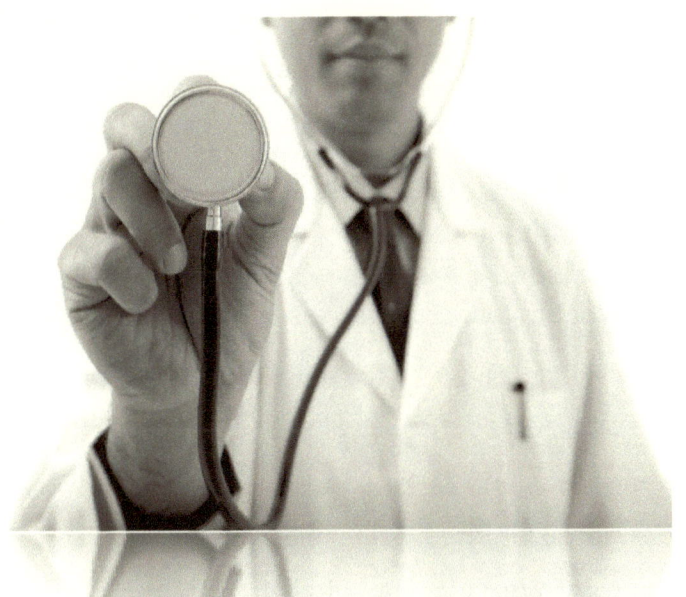

Let me elucidate shortly why I came to write this guide to integral, holistic health.

It was not out of sheer curiosity, nor for attracting readers to my rather voluminous book collection. Instead, my *primary motivation* was that during all of my childhood and youth, not only myself, but also my mother, grandmother, and later my wife were to suffer *medical malpractice*.

I can say with conviction that my mother had lived at least ten years longer, had she not trusted the ignorance of the gods in white coats, or what I came to call *'international medical business.'*

My wife was almost killed by a doctor who had performed a spinal punctation with local anesthesia, for which it is absolutely paramount that the patient be in a *horizontal position* for at least twenty-four hours, without interruption.

What the doctor did was to send my wife home after a few hours. The result was that she had to be hospitalized as she was almost dying from the headaches and other consequences of this very dangerous intervention. I was interviewing several doctors in our local hospital about her case and one of them was scandalized and said that the operation had been a clear case of medical malpractice. But a moment later, when I said I was a law student and intended to sue that doctor for medical malpractice, and wanted him to testify in court against his colleague, he waved me off, saying I had

WHY DID I WRITE THIS GUIDE?

'misunderstood' him and that he could not allege anything of the kind.

Two minutes later I was out of the office. Needless to add that he had not invited me to come back.

I became aware what a sordid club this modern medicine was, how false and sworn into stubborn resistance these doctors were, and I began to understand that they had indeed much to lose and much to defend, that namely their whole brilliant empire was built on very shaky ground.

That same year, suffering from hemorrhoids, I submitted to an 'operation' suggested by a doctor in the nearby hospital. It was a torture, no other words can be used for describing it. Already during the examination, the doctor with his Nazi haircut (and attitude) hurt me badly by flapping apart my anus without using any lubricant, and the hurt was worse because he used a rubber glove. That should have given me a 'foreplay' to what I was going to experience during the operation, which consisted in inserting a huge phallic tampon, almost as thick as a beer bottle, into my anus while under anesthesia. The waking up, and gradual vanishing of the aesthetics was extremely painful, despite the pain killers I got. I had to stay three entire days and nights with this monstrous device in my anus.

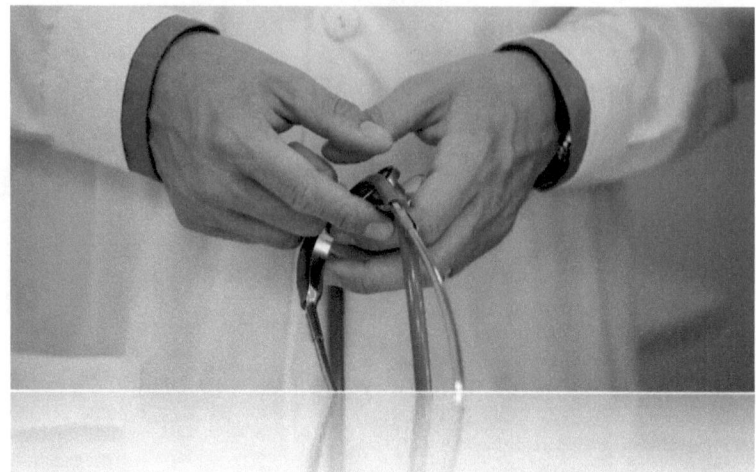

The explanation those mechanistic doctor-robots gave me and my mother was that my sphincter had been 'too tight' and had therefore to be 'opened.' That was being done, and so well that during any even slight diarrhea I get it all into the bed. And as to 'curing' the hemorrhoids, the result was that it all got worse. The operation took place when I was 18-years old. I am 60 now and while I myself found a solution to curing hemorrhoids later in life, I suffer from the additional 'side-effect' of the operation that I cannot withhold my feces during sleep and when I have diarrhea as this happens ever so often when living in South-East Asia.

WHY DID I WRITE THIS GUIDE?

So what was this torture-operation good for other than giving 'medical business' to the doctors and the hospital? And to stay with the hemorrhoid problem for a moment, and taking it as an example, I finally did my own research what actually causes hemorrhoids in the first place. It has nothing to do with the 'tightness' of the sphincter, to begin with. A good sphincter should be tight for that's its function after all. Does that make sense to you? It may, but it doesn't for that matter make sense to doctor-idiots who are brainwashed into 'medical business' and apply concepts that are making money, not concepts that heal people.

Second, hemorrhoids are largely the result of wrong diet. At that time, at age 18, I was eating lots of red meat which is about the worst you can do to your body in terms of food, for red meat takes a very long time to digest while our intestines are not made for eating meat. They are relatively long compared to read meat eaters such as tigers or lions. These animals namely have a short intestinal tract, thus the meat won't stay too long in there and rot there to a stinking mass of debris in fermentation. Take a gorilla, on the other hand, a vegetarian; these animals have long intestines such as human beings. That's one of many examples that show that humans should be vegetarians, as a matter of biology! (No need to come up with 'spiritual do's and dont's).

Third, I was still ingesting lots of Western pharmaceuticals in my youth, many of which have a negative effect upon the growth of hemorrhoids because they are outright acidic. It's when the stool gets too acidic that the condition of the entire body changes 'polarity' and becomes potential sickness-attractor.

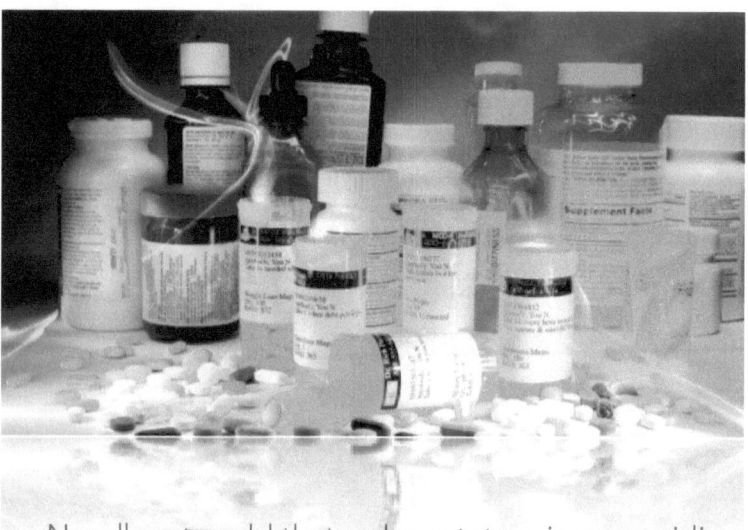

Needless to add that red meat, too, is very acidic.

—See Dr. Robert O. Young, The pH Miracle: Balance Your Diet, Reclaim Your Health (2010), Dr. N.W. Walker, the Natural Way to Vibrant Health (1972), Dr. George Watson,

WHY DID I WRITE THIS GUIDE?

Nutrition and Your Mind: The Psychochemical Response (1972), Dr. Maoshing Ni, The Tao of Nutrition (2012).

Now, to close this chapter, there is well a happy end, but only through my own smart. Since I am a full vegetarian, and even though I am sometimes smoking cigars, I have no more problem with hemorrhoids. I could have got there without the nonsensical 'operation' as I still have the side-effect of it in terms of my anal sphincter being too loose now. Hence, the whole medical diagnosis was wrong, from the first to the last point. And I was not properly informed about the noxious effects and the utter pain that this operation would cause. The doctor did not fully inform me, and this is how it goes in most cases!

Not only that most doctors in the West have no what really causes disease, what most upset me is how sluggishly most doctors handle their obligation to get the patient's full consent for any treatment they engage. In practice namely, doctors take it for granted that the patient gives his consent, with the difference however that this consent is not an informed one because the patient has in the regular case not been properly informed what the treatment really incurs, short term, and in the long run.

ALTERNATIVE MEDICINE AND WELLNESS TECHNIQUES

After all, my mother was virtually killed by those doctors in the Catholic hospital where she was constantly maltreated and sadly died at an age when she did not need to, only because the doctors did not recognize the psychic condition of her heart disease and virtually massacred her, by one operation after the other, until her heart was stuffed with metal machinery—that her body eventually rejected!

These shortcomings got me to be interested in *alternative medicine* from about my thirties. I first had the opportunity to study Reiki with Anneke van Gelder, a *Reiki Master* from Holland, acquiring the first degree, then, five years later, with Chandra Naidu from South Africa, acquiring the second degree or initiation in the Usui alternative healing system. The third, and most important initiation, which results in the title of *Reiki Master*, was offered to me by Ugo di Marino, an Italian *Reiki Master*, in Bali, in 2000, but I refused to receive it, as I felt I was not ready.

WHY DID I WRITE THIS GUIDE?

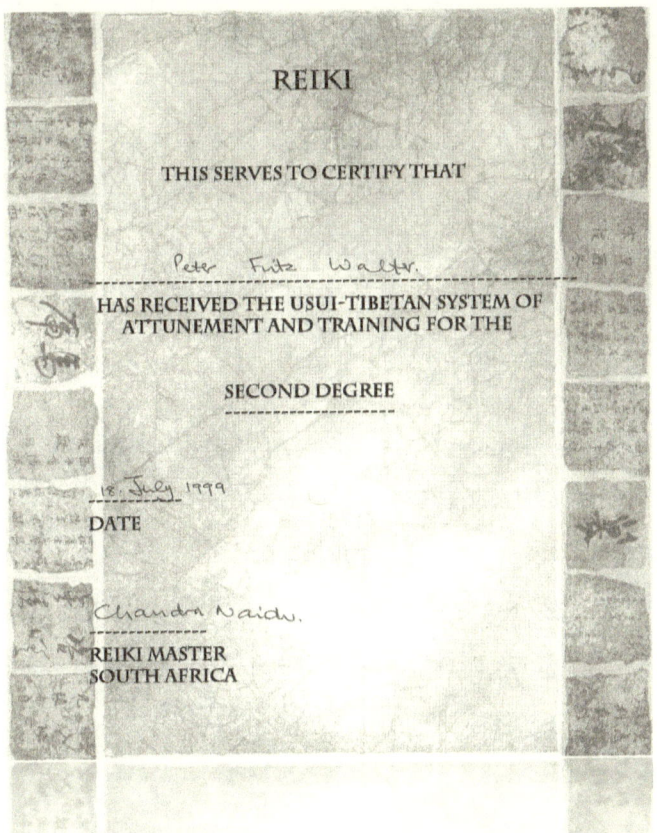

Ugo had waived the twenty thousand dollars fee that is obligatory for receiving this title, and I didn't find it correct to receive the title without giving 'money energy' back for the energy received. In addition, I felt I wasn't dedicated enough, at that time, distracted by a quite important business project.

But this *Reiki Master* told me I had all the capacities of a true master in this art of energy healing. The most important feedback I got from Anneke, back in 1994, when I started out with my Reiki practice. Anneke had quite a number of students, and a thriving practice, with patients from the middle and upper classes in Rotterdam. Anneke was a very gifted healer; she was able to do distance healing as well. Some of her patients were Americans whom she treated over the phone, at any time of the day or the night, however the client found it convenient.

Now for me, as I never had done any healing practice and had no idea I had a talent for it, it was important what Anneke could sense when I treated her, after having learnt the basics. And surprisingly so, Anneke said I was an exceptional student, that she never had somebody with just beginner knowledge who had such a powerful energy body.

Only later was I informed by potential astrology that, besides having Sun in the 6th House, which is the quintessential 'healer' positioning of the Sun in a birth chart, I was having quite a few constellations in my chart that were pointing to my talent for healing and my strong luminous energy field.

Finally, between 1998 and 2000, being a member of the *Parapsychological Association* of Jakarta, Indonesia, I was screened by several first rate psychics who fully confirmed what Anneke had told me. The

WHY DID I WRITE THIS GUIDE?

psychics said that my human energy field was exceptionally strong and powerful and that I should use it for healing others. And a test was made. Several boys who had been circumcised were taken to me for treatment and the results were convincing and surprising everybody, including the boys' fathers who were attending the healing session.

What I did was simply to hold both of my hands about 5 inches over the penis of a boy, for about half an hour, ejecting energy from my palms, which was felt by the boys as 'warm and nice.'

One boy was dreadfully maltreated by the quack who had cut his foreskin. He was still bleeding after one week and his penis looked painfully distorted. It was all inflamed and the boy, according to what his father said, suffered from his condition more than any other boy. He suffered atrocious pain when urinating.

This boy I treated twice, on two consecutive mornings, each time for about one hour, and the results were miraculous. After the first treatment, the boy was pain-free and could urinate without pain. And the bleeding stopped right after the treatment. After the second treatment, the boy smiled, for the first time, and said:

ALTERNATIVE MEDICINE AND WELLNESS TECHNIQUES

—I feel good now, I think it's all good.

After my long stay in Indonesia, I was suffering from an ongoing diarrhea and upon returning back to Germany, I was seeing a *Reiki Master*. She had been initiated by powerful Filipino healers in the Philippines. Again, I got to hear I had been the victim of medical malpractice because the diagnosis by her husband, a medical doctor, revealed that my intestinal flora was completely gone. The doctor was scandalized, saying:

— You have no more bacteria in your intestines, so how is your body going to digest any food? It's impossible. We have to rebuild your intestinal flora, and that will take some time. Until then, you need to be on a strict diet.

I had been consulting Western doctors in Jakarta who had given me huge amounts of antibiotics, and as my condition was recurring, I took those antibiotics almost for one whole year. My condition was healed completely, only through homeopathy, Bach Flowers and Reiki, and later on, upon returning to Asia, with Chinese herbal concoctions. And the third motivational factor, then, for my research on alternative medicine and wellness techniques was

WHY DID I WRITE THIS GUIDE?

what I was learning about native healing in Indonesia first, and then, a few years later in Vietnam and Cambodia.

When I first arrived in Yogyakarta, back in 1996, I remember to have counted between 120 and 150 shops and street kiosks that were selling the age-old *Jamu* plant medicine, and related homeopathic products of which the local culture in Java used to be so rich. Jamu is a yellow powder that is won from grinding the roots of certain trees. This powder, then, is mixed with hot water and the yellow of an egg, and this gives a cup of delicious brew that heals about everything. There were more than one hundred different Jamu concoctions in one of the larger shops.

The street kiosks were selling between five and twenty of them, sufficient for the common ailments such as 'sakit panas' (fever), 'diare' (diarrhea), or 'anak-anak panas' (child fever).

In fact, fever is a severe and very dangerous condition in Java and also in Bali. I have spoken to a young man who lost his two small children in one night. The fever was shooting up so quickly that every help was too late. These two small babies died and left behind a couple in deep and lasting depression.

ALTERNATIVE MEDICINE AND WELLNESS TECHNIQUES

Of course, in such a case, Western medicine could have helped effectively, but the man was very poor and I am not sure he could have afforded to pay the hospital.

Two years later, I was shocked to see that only about ten to twenty of those shops and kiosks remained, and a year later, in 1999, I was counting just five. Why had all the others disappeared? It was because of Western medicine suddenly being recognized as 'better' and 'cleaner,' and so on and so forth, through television and USA-driven publicity. It appeared that only people in the countryside, and elders, were keeping true to their traditional medicine.

The problem is complex. Pharmacies I saw in Indonesia, Vietnam and Cambodia sell Western pharmaceutical products like bread, without any product knowledge, and any restriction. All can be bought that is in-store, no prescription needed. As these locals cannot read the leaflets, they have hardly any knowledge about the particular pharmaceuticals, and their side-effects and dangers.

Both in Saigon, Vietnam and in Phnom Penh, Cambodia I have seen in several shops *Valium 20* that

WHY DID I WRITE THIS GUIDE?

since decades is legally forbidden in Europe, sold to a teenager.

The prices are much higher compared to the very cheap Jamu concoctions. Jamu typically was sold for about ten cent per concoction, while for most medicines, it used to be a few dollars each, but now has gotten much more expensive, so expensive namely that locals who are simple workers or rice farmers—and that is about 80% of the Cambodian population, with a salary of 2 dollars/day—cannot afford them.

So there are *two problem complexes* interwoven with each other. The first is lack of knowledge. While the Jamu sellers had excellent knowledge of their products, this is seldom the case with modern-day pharmacies, in these countries. The second problem is the financial hurdle, as modern pharmacy virtually bleeds the locals out, who in urgent cases take exorbitant credits with village usurers, for which they pay *between twenty and sixty percent* of monthly (not yearly) interest!

With hospitals, it's the same. In Cambodia, when somebody has not enough money to pay the doctor upon arrival in the hospital, the person is not treated.

ALTERNATIVE MEDICINE AND WELLNESS TECHNIQUES

I have heard many stories of people who died virtually under the eyes of doctors because they had not enough money to pay for an urgency operation. So they were not treated.

Back in 2005, a Vietnamese friend of mine in Cambodia was having an unwanted pregnancy but did not opt for abortion. When the baby was on the point to come out, she quickly went to a hospital and called me to send her two hundred dollars for paying the doctor. I replied that it was okay and that I was sending the money with my driver, who however came to be stuck in a traffic jam.

The doctor refused to help the baby to leave the womb as the money had not arrived in time, and the baby died in the womb and had to be removed surgically. The doctor cashed the two hundred dollars in for giving birth to a dead fetus.

Another consequence of medical costs, that is even uglier than this story, is a fact that was reported to me by several trustworthy university graduates. In Cambodia, when a person is injured by a traffic accident, the hospital costs might be outrageous for a local person who has caused the accident. The simple and brutal consequence is that victims are killed and

WHY DID I WRITE THIS GUIDE?

those who are guilty of causing the accident take it and leave it.

In one case, witnessed by a friend of mine, a trustworthy business graduate, a truck driver had collided with a motorcycle, and the heavily injured and bleeding woman who drove the motorcycle was screaming, on the floor, a few meters in front of the truck. The driver did not think long, restarted the motor, drove right over the screaming victim, and took flight.

When police and ambulance arrived, every help was too late. I was told that this happens in Phnom Penh virtually every day. The reason is not a particular murderous instinct in Cambodian people, but the outrageous hospital costs and absence of any obligatory national insurance.

I recently had my maid's uncle being hospitalized for a stroke. The doctors didn't do anything as the family is very poor. The moment they knew I was willing to pay, several doctors came to examine the man. Subsequently, an x-ray was proposed that was quoted to me with two hundred dollars while locals normally pay between twenty and thirty dollars for the same x-ray. It's all a question of money, the whole medical business, and that is why I call it so. *It is a business, and nothing but a business!* And its objective is *not healing*, but money-making.

It is significant that for Western doctors, the expression 'healer' is an insult. They should be called medical business consultants, or pharmaceutical sales agents for that's what they are.

AYURVEDA

The Science of Life

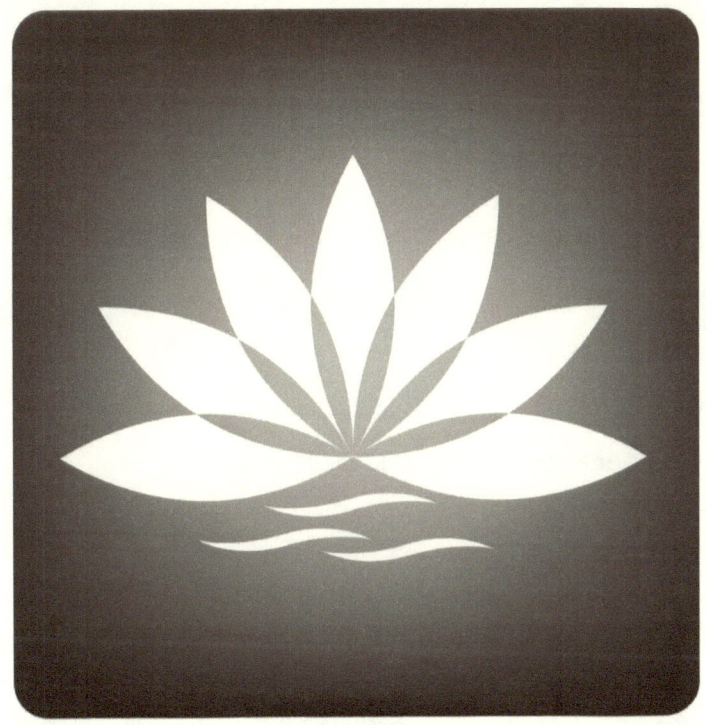

I was becoming aware of Ayurveda when, back in the 1970s, I was reading Gandhi. Gandhi was often reporting in his writings that he put his faith not in modern medicine but in age-old Ayurveda and that he had healed all his ailments with the simple food recipes for healthy living that Ayurveda teaches as a matter of prophylaxis.

I was intrigued and bought a book about Ayurveda and the information resonated deeply in my soul. I found many of the Ayurveda precepts very similar to what I had learnt about Chinese and Tibetan Medicine.

The name *Ayurveda* is significant as it means something like *Life Knowledge* or *Science of Life*—and there is about no greater gap to traditional Western medicine which could be called *Science of Death* because it gained knowledge not from observing the living changes in life's texture, but by vivisecting cadavers.

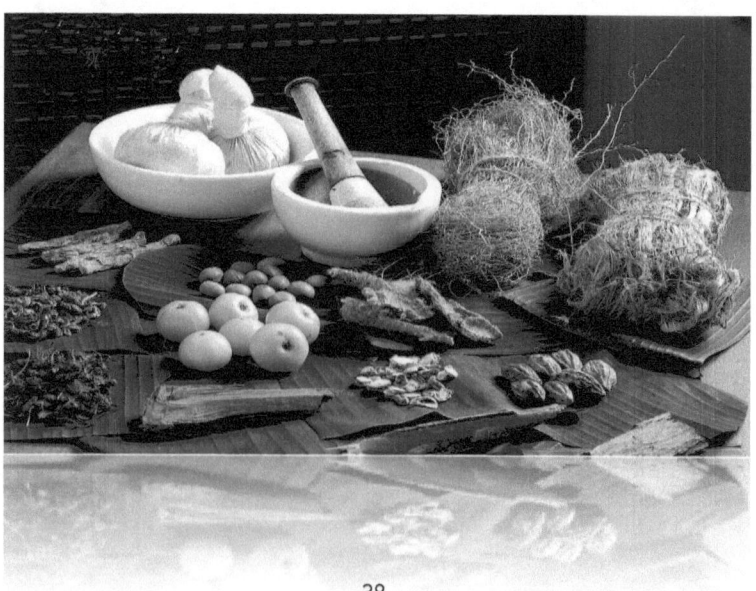

WHY DID I WRITE THIS ARTICLE?

Ayurveda deals with the measures of *healthy living,* along with therapeutic measures that relate to physical, mental, social and spiritual harmony. Ayurveda is also one among the few traditional systems of medicine involving surgery.

Ayurveda is a wholeness and wellness approach to medicine which means that *its concepts are holistic* and consider life as a dynamic process. It avoids any harsh and especially irrevocable treatments and favors *soft remedies* such as plant concoctions, and massage. On a trip to India back in 2006, I was having Ayurveda treatments in a reputed *Ayurveda Clinic* in Trivandrum, Kerala. I got daily massage with warm oil, which is a wonderful therapy that relaxed me deeply. After the first treatments, before I got used to it, I was so completely relaxed and put at rest, that upon coming back to the hotel, I had to sleep for the entire afternoon.

One day, I took an additional treatment, thus after the massage, that they call steam bath, but it's not like a steam sauna at all. You are sitting in a wooden container to which a tube is connected that transports the hot vapor. The casing is closed around you and there is a rubber ring around your neck that prevents steam from getting out. So your face and head are cold while your body gets very hot, and that is a wise idea.

    I was sitting in that wooden box, on a little chair, and saw in front of me a stove on which a water kettle was boiling. From the top of the kettle there was that tube leading right to a pipe system that borders the bottom of the box. There are many little holes in these pipes from which the vapor streams into the box.

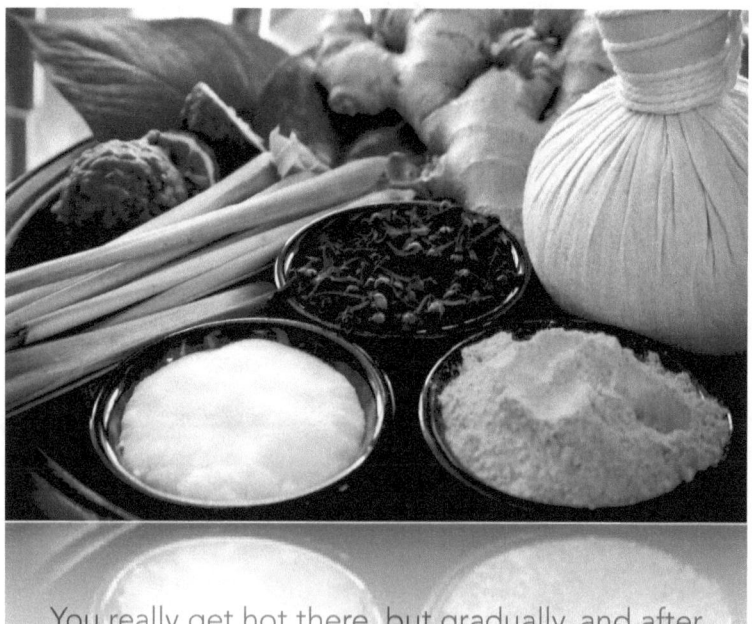

    You really get hot there, but gradually, and after fifteen minutes, just at the right moment, they liberate you from this sweating experience. And the surprise

WHY DID I WRITE THIS ARTICLE?

was that that day, when I came back to the hotel, I was not tired at all.

I never knew that a steam bath can revitalize you to that extent! And yes, I forgot to mention the most important. It's not just vapor but in that kettle were a lot of fresh herbs boiling in the water …

Then I went to an Ayurveda doctor and got some medicine against diarrhea and another one for my swelling legs. But unfortunately I had to leave the whole plastic bag at the airport in Trivandrum because they really take flight safety serious in India, to a point to annoy you, and only one bag is allowed to take on-board, and I had already two with me, and my suitcase was full to a breaking point …, so I had to leave all that wonderful medicine behind in India.

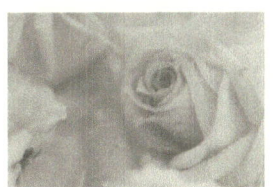

Traditional Chinese Medicine

Another Life Science

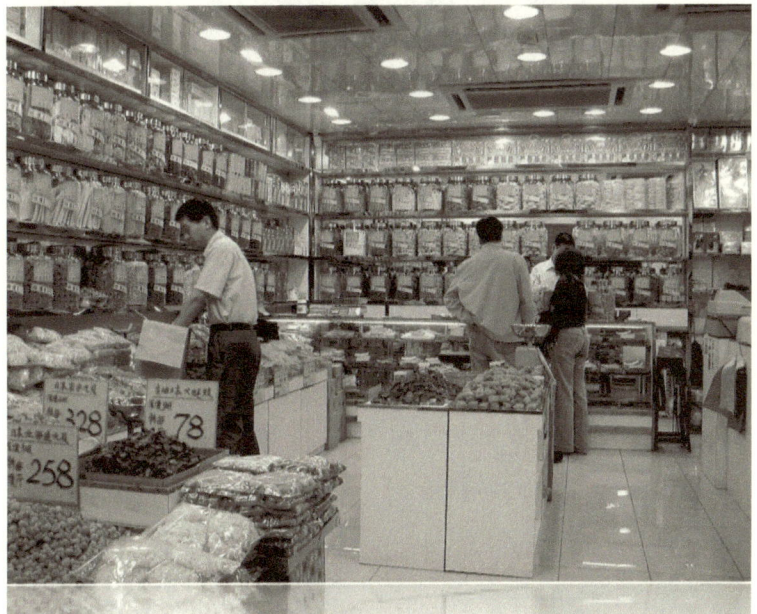

Traditional Chinese medicine is a range of traditional medical practices used in China that developed over several thousand years. These practices include herbal medicine, acupuncture, and massage.

Other East Asian medical systems, such as traditional Japanese, Korean or Tibetan medicine, apply similar principles.

Chinese medicine was perhaps the first really *holistic* medicine on the globe, and it sees processes of the human body as interrelated and constantly interacting energetically with the environment.

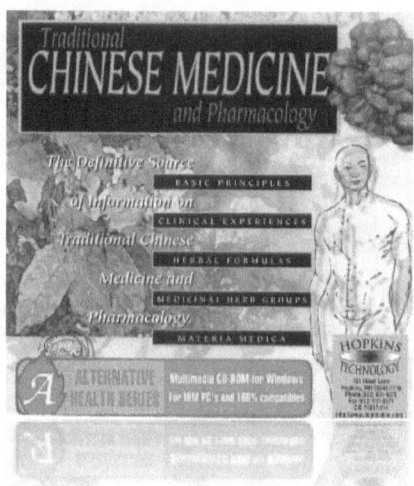

Chinese medicine recognizes that good health is basically a state of harmony and therefore looks for the *signs of disharmony* in the external and internal environment of a person in order to understand, treat and prevent disease.

It was back in the 1980s that I got to learn about Chinese Medicine for the first time. I was reading several books about it and discovered a truly holistic approach to health, something completely unknown until this day to palliative and symptom-focused Western 'business' medicine.

As I set out to study it more in detail, I found, in 1995, a CD-ROM produced by Hopkins University with the title *Traditional Chinese Medicine and Pharmacology*, from which I will provide some quotes here. The author is the Director of the All-China Association of Traditional Chinese Medicine and Advisor to the Public Health Ministry of the People's Republic of China, Professor Don Jianhua:

> The basic theories of traditional Chinese medicine describe the physiology and pathology of the human body, disease etiology, diagnosis, and differentiation of symptom-complexes. This includes the theories of Yin-Yang, Five Elements, zang-fu, channels-collaterals, qi, blood, body fluid, methods of diagnosis, and differentiation of symptom-complexes.
>
> Traditional Chinese medical theories possess two outstanding features, their holistic point of view, and their application of treatment according to the differentiation of symptom-complexes. According to these traditional viewpoints, the zang-fu organs are the core of the human body as an organic entity in which tissues and sense organs are connected through a network of channels and collaterals. This concept is applied extensively to physiology, pathology, diagnosis, and treatment.

The functional physiological activities of the zang-fu organs are dissimilar, but they work in coordination. There exists an organic connection between the organs and their related tissues. Pathologically, a dysfunction of the zang-fu organs may be reflected on the body surface through the channels and their collaterals. At the same time, diseases of body surface tissues may also affect their related zang or fu organs. Affected zang or fu organs may also influence each other through internal connections. Traditional Chinese medical treatment consists of regulating the functions of the zang-fu organs in order to correct pathological changes. With acupuncture, treatment is accomplished by stimulating certain areas of the external body.

Not only is the human body an organic whole, but it is also a unified entity within nature, so changes in the natural environment may directly or indirectly affect it. For example, changes of the four seasons, and the alternations of day and night may change the functional condition of the human body, while various geographical environments can influence differences in body constitution, and so on. These factors must be considered when diagnosis and treatment are given. The principles of treatment are expected to accord with the different seasons and environments.

Application of treatment according to the differentiation of syndromes is another characteristic of traditional Chinese medicine. 'Differentiation of syndromes' means to analyze the disease condition in order to know its essentials, to identify the causative facts, the location and nature, and to obtain conclusions about the confrontation between pathogenic and antipathogenic factors.

TRADITIONAL CHINESE MEDICINE

In traditional Chinese medicine, differentiation performed to outline the specific principles and methods of treatment because similar diseases may have different clinical manifestations, while different diseases may share the same syndromes.

Treatment in traditional Chinese medicine stresses the differences of syndromes, but not the differences of diseases. Therefore different treatments for the same disease exist and different diseases can be treated by the same method.

— Copyright 2005 Hopkins Technology

This opened me doors to a more thorough understanding of the particular approach of Chinese traditional medicine to restoring health as well as to disease prevention. There is namely a much stronger focus in Chinese medicine upon *disease prevention* as this is the case in Western medicine.

The primordial energy, when working on the earth plane, manifests in dualistic form, as two complementary energies, *Yin and Yang*. Both of the energies can be associated with certain characteristics. *Yin* can be associated with the female principle; this does however not mean that it is identical with it. We talk about corresponding characteristics or elements, and the system as such is one of corresponding relationships. Accordingly, *yin* can be said to correspond with water, the female principle, the color black, the direction down or a landscape that is flat. *Yang* can be said to correspond with fire, the male principle, the color white, the direction up or with a landscape that is mountainous. In every *yin* there is a bit of *yang*, and in every *yang* a bit of *yin*.

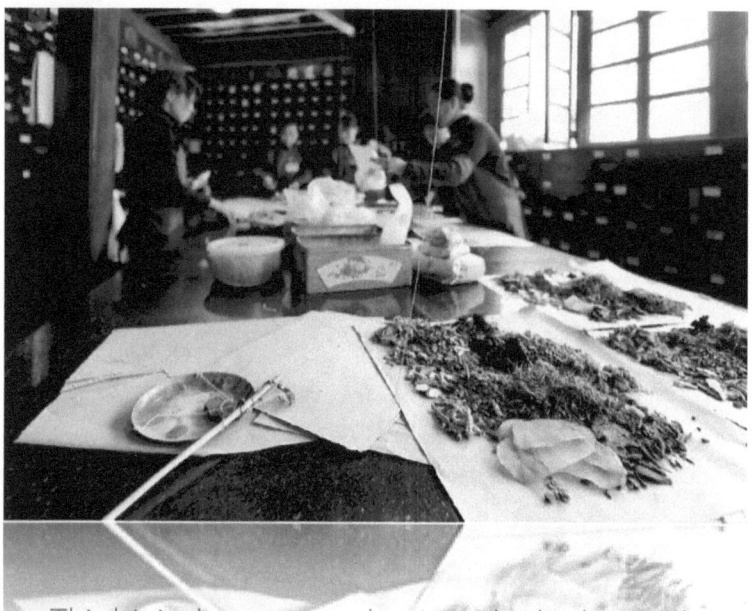

This bit is the essence that is multiplied once the point of culmination has been passed. Professor Don Jianhua writes:

> Yin and yang represent two opposite aspects of every object and its implicit conflict and interdependence. Generally, anything that is moving, ascending, bright,

TRADITIONAL CHINESE MEDICINE

progressing, hyperactive, including functional disease of the body, pertains to yang. The characteristics of stillness, descending, darkness, degeneration, hypoactivity, including organic disease, pertain to yin.

The nature of yin and yang is relative. According to Yin-Yang theory, everything in the universe can be divided into the two opposite but complementary aspects of yin and yang and so on ad infinitum. For example, day is yang and night is yin, but morning is understood as being yang within yang, afternoon is yin within yang, evening before midnight is yin within yin and the time after midnight is yang within yin.

— Copyright 2005 Hopkins Technology

What that means is that for example *yin* moves towards its fullness in order to culminate and swap its nature into *yang*. *Yang*, when it culminates, becomes *yin*. That is why we can say change is programmed into the very essence of the *yin-yang* dualism and thus, change cannot be avoided. We can even go as far as saying that the very fact of change is the proof that we deal with a living thing. If there is no change, there is no movement and, as a result, no life. Life is change, living movement.

The *yin-yang* duality principle is very far-reaching. It also encompasses the art of cooking. The Tao of cooking prescribes that every dish should be composed in a way to balance *yin* and *yang* and the four tastes sweet, salty, sour and bitter. Every vegetable, every kind of meat or fish, and every other food has been qualified by the sages of old to be either *yin* or *yang*.

This knowledge forms an essential part of the Chinese system of health care and of the martial arts, which can be expressed in the slogan 'food is medicine.' Professor Don Jianhua explains:

> The yin and yang aspects within an object are not quiescent, but in a state of constant motion. They can be described as being in a state where the lessening of yin leads to an increase of yang, or vice versa. (...)
>
> Regarding the human body's functional activities, which are considered yang, the consumption of nutrient substances which are considered yin, results in the lessening of yin to the increase of yang. As the metabolism of nutrient substances (yin) exhausts the functional energy (yang) to a certain extent, this is understood as a lessening of yang to the increase of yin. Under normal conditions the mutual consuming and increasing of yin and yang maintain a relative balance. Under abnormal conditions there is an excess or insufficiency of either yin or yang which leads to the occurrence of disease.
>
> — Copyright 2005 Hopkins Technology

TRADITIONAL CHINESE MEDICINE

In the martial arts, the same principle applies. The beginner of learning the art of Kung Fu is developing consciousness. And second breathing. The right way of breathing stresses that we exhale on the effort.

It is not the muscles that do exceptional things, but breath or *prana*. In Kung Fu exercises the perfection of the movements is impossible to achieve if the breathing technique is wrong. You can even say that the movements have no value in themselves except forcing us to breathe correctly.

By balancing *yin* and *yang* in our mindbody, the very source of our being, the Tao within us becomes activated and can more easily guide us and enrich us from inside. It is our true power. But without balancing *yin* and *yang* in our mindbody, its power is spoilt by the many negative influences that modern life inflicts upon it.

Our emotions, like all in life, are reigned by the *duality principle*, they ebb up and they flow down, they increase and they decrease, and eventually they go through a culmination point and then change.

ALTERNATIVE MEDICINE AND WELLNESS TECHNIQUES

Let me demonstrate this again with an example. When you are enraged, your rage will increase until it reaches a culmination point.

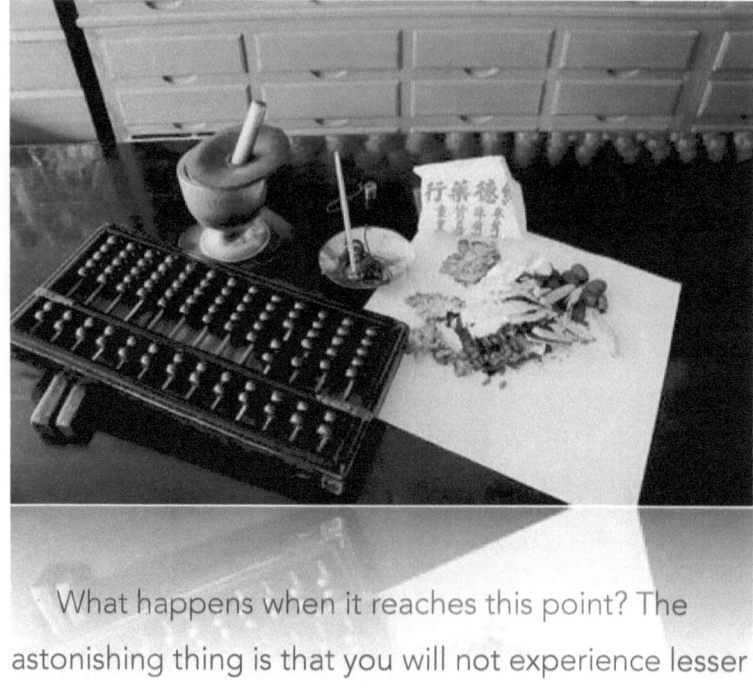

What happens when it reaches this point? The astonishing thing is that you will not experience lesser rage then, but no rage at all!

Your rage will change into another emotion, for example joy, or it will completely cease with no other emotion overtaking: you are at peace.

Why is that so? This is so because all our emotions are interconnected in what I call a *kaleidoscopic succession*. A kaleidoscope is a device where the prism is split off by a lens into its basic spectral colors.

TRADITIONAL CHINESE MEDICINE

These devices that many of us know from our childhood, are designed like little photographic cameras or glasses and you could look at any object using the kaleidoscope as a filter. You would then see life in many different colorful shades. This metaphor fits emotions very well.

Our emotions are the basic spectral colors of the light beam of life which is like a bundled beam of white light. Every emotion, by the frequency of the spectral color that it adds on to the beam of the bioenergy, completes the white beam. As you know from optics, light can only be white if the spectrum is complete.

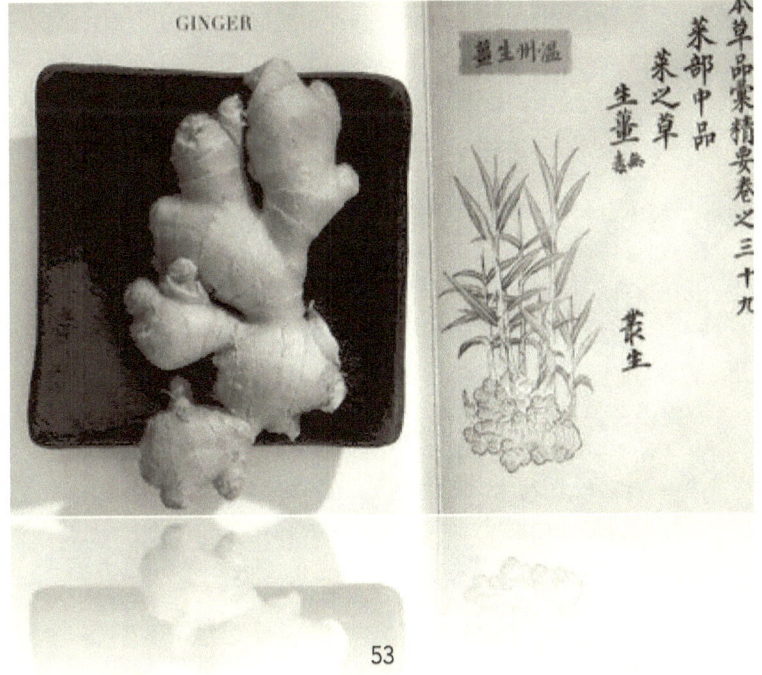

And so it is with our emotions. Your vital energies are only complete and strong if all your emotions are active and contribute their specific bioelectric frequencies to the main frequency of the bioenergy that flows through your organism.

When you block one of the emotions, that part of the frequency is lacking or becomes distorted. As a result, your white beam of vital energy will not be really white anymore and thus will be weakened. That is why the duality of our emotions is so important and must be functional if emotions are to flow healthily.

Now, let us see who this interrelatedness and mutual transformation of yin and yang which could also be called the 'dualistic principle' works in the holistic treatment of disease. Professor Don Jianhua writes:

> The mutual transformation of yin and yang is often seen during the development of a disease. For example, if a patient has a constant high fever, which is suddenly lowered, accompanied by a pale complexion, cold limbs, extremely feeble pulse (the danger symptoms of yin cold syndromes), we may say that the disease has transformed from a yang syndrome into a yin syndrome. Under these circumstances, proper emergency treatment should warm the limbs to make the pulse normal. The yang qi will recover, and the

danger will be removed. Thus yin syndromes can change into yang syndromes. (…)

For example, the activities (yang) of a particular organ are based on that organ's substance (yin) and when either of these aspects are absent, the other cannot function. Thus the result of physiological activities is to constantly promote the transformation of yang into yin essence. If yin and yang cannot maintain relative balance and interaction, they will separate from each other ending the life that depends on them. (…)

In medical treatment, the theory of yin and yang is not only used to decide the principles of treatment. This theory is also generally applied to the properties, flavor and action of Chinese herbal medicine as a guide to the clinical administration of herbs. For example, drugs with cold, cool or moist properties are classified as yin and drugs with the opposite properties are classified as yang. Herbs with sour, bitter, or salty flavors are yin, while those with pungent, sweet, or insipid flavors are yang. Drugs with an astringent or descending action are yin and those with an ascending and dispersing action are yang. In clinical treatment, we should determine the principles of treatment based on an analysis of the yin and yang conditions present in terms of their different yin-yang properties and actions. The goal of clinical treatment is to restore the healthy yin-yang properties and actions to restore a healthy yin-yang balance in the patient.

—Copyright 2005 Hopkins Technology

The *principle of the five elements* suggests that nature is *interactive* and in a continuous process of transformation. The five elements wood, fire, water, earth and metal are mutually constructive and also mutually destructive.

For example, wood is positively enhanced by water whereas water destroys fire. These two parallel processes of creation and destruction can be seen as two circles or cycles, a *cycle of creation*, and a *cycle of destruction*. Professor Don Jianhua explains the five elements theory in these terms:

> The Five Elements theory posits wood, fire, earth, metal, and water as the basic elements of the material world. These elements are in constant movement and change. Moreover, the complex connections between material objects are explained through the relationship of interdependence and mutual restraint that governs the five elements. In traditional Chinese medicine Five Elements Theory is used to interpret the relationship between the physiology and pathology of the human body and the natural environment.
>
> — Copyright 2005 Hopkins Technology

The principle of the five elements teaches us that nothing in nature is static or stagnant, but that all is subject to continuous flow, continuous change. It also teaches us that all elements naturally interact with each other, mutually depend on each other, and that nothing is really isolated. As a result, we can verify if our understanding of nature is in accordance with the laws of nature.

Studying and observing these laws, we notice a high degree of *interdependence* in nature and a high *interactivity*, a fact that in the Western sciences has only recently been given the focus it deserves. It is modern systems theory that deals with the interactive processes in nature.

> —See Fritjof Capra, The Web of Life (1997), The Hidden Connections (2002), and The Systems View of Life (2014).

The principle of the *five elements*, as simplistic as it may seem on first sight, is a wonderful teacher of real-life functions that can help us to correct our way to see the world, ourselves and others and to more accurately evaluate the impact that every single of our actions might have on life as a whole. It is the point of departure of a holistic view of life. Professor Don Jianhua writes:

> The Five Elements theory is applied to the physiology and pathology of the human body by using the relationship of generation and subjugation to guide clinical diagnosis and treatment. (…)

Physiologically the Five Elements theory explains the unity of the mutual relationships between the zang-fu organs and body tissues as well as between the human body and nature. The physiological activities of the five zang organs can be classified according to the different characteristics of the five elements. For example, the liver is said to preside over the vigorous flow of qi and also has the function of ensuring free qi circulation. Since these characteristics are similar to the properties of wood, the liver is categorized as wood in the scheme of the five elements. Heart yang has a warming action so it belongs to the category of the fire element. The spleen is the source of transformation of essential substances and is associated with the earth element's characteristics of growth and transformation. The lung has clearing and descending properties and is associated with the metal element's characteristics of clearing and astringency. The kidney has the function of controlling water metabolism and storing essence and is associated with the water element's characteristics of moistening and flowing downward.

— Copyright 2005 Hopkins Technology

Our emotions are *interactive* in two ways, they interact with each other and they interact with the environment, with other people's emotions and even with surrounding natural energies such as the weather. Yes, our emotions influence the weather; this is not a superstition but one of the age-old wisdom teachings that Wilhelm Reich's *orgone research* has corroborated.

TRADITIONAL CHINESE MEDICINE

Vice versa, the macrocosmic energies contained in the earth atmosphere, and even solar spots influence our emotions.

There is nothing really separated in nature. All of us know the disastrous influence negative people can have over a mass audience.

Homeopathy

From Paracelsus to Masaru Emoto

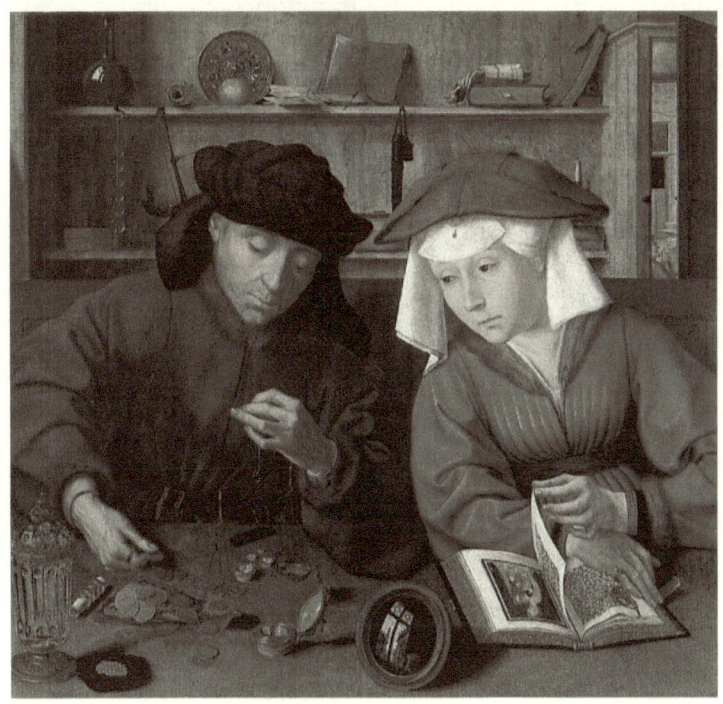

Introduction

In the following sub-chapters about Paracelsus, Samuel Hahnemann, Edward Bach and Masaru Emoto, I shall explain in detail how I came to try and use homeopathy and how wonderfully it helped to cure an almost fatal disease that was brought about by a continuous and irresponsible medical prescription of antibiotics against recurring diarrhea.

The most important general principle of homeopathy is that it restores the natural *yin-yang* balance in the organism by restoring the vital energy flow, and it does this by etheric substances that are dissolved in water, thereby using the *hado*, the memory of water, to hold on to the specific vibrations and transmit them to the client who drinks the water.

I would like to recommend to the reader the following publications, all of which I have not only studied but also reviewed. The links lead directly to my book reviews.

Donna Eden

Energy Medicine (1999)
The Energy Medicine Kit (2004)

Masaru Emoto

The Hidden Messages in Water (2004)
The Secret Life of Water (2005)

Richard Gerber

A Guide to Vibrational Medicine (2001)

Shafica Karagulla

The Chakras (1989)

ERVIN LASZLO
Science and the Akashic Field (2004)

LYNNE MCTAGGART
The Field (2002)

PARACELSUS

I read *Paracelsus (1493–1541)*, whose real name was *Theophrastus Philippus Aureolus Bombastus von Hohenheim* rather early in life, at the time when I was reading Franz Anton Mesmer, back in 1975, when I enrolled in law school at age twenty. And I saw the similarity between the two otherwise very different personalities, regarding their discovery of the bioplasmatic energy, or *human energy field*.

Paracelsus truly was a holistic healer. He continued an ancient tradition that for the majority in his time was completely lost. It was the *Hermetic Healing Tradition*. It must be noted that the breakup with this holistic healing tradition occurred not after the downfall of the Greek Empire, but in the midst of it. It was *Hippocrates*, often cited as the great medical benefactor of humanity, who was actually the greatest detractor of true healing. Manly P. Hall writes in *The*

Secret Teachings of All Ages (1928/2003) about Hippocrates that he was the one single physician who, during the fifth century before Christ dissociated the healing arts from the other sciences of the temple and thereby established a precedent of separateness. Hall pursues:

> One of the consequences is the present widespread crass scientific materialism. The ancients realized the interdependence of the sciences. The moderns do not; and as a result, incomplete systems of learning are attempting to maintain isolated individualism. The obstacles which confront present-day scientific research are largely the result of prejudicial limitations imposed by those who are unwilling to accept that which transcends the concrete perceptions of the five primary human senses.
>
> — Manly P. Hall, The Secret Teachings of All Ages (1928/2003), 344.

Below I will provide some more details about this tradition and how Paracelsus applied it in his own holistic approach to healing.

But I would like to begin with the beginning, the starting principle of life as it were, that after all was never ever recognized in the West as a scientifically provable principle or pattern in both the macro—and the microcosm.

HOMEOPATHY

This principle or pattern is the *human energy field*, or cosmic life energy.

Paracelsus discovered this force everywhere, and both in the plant and animal realm, and he called it *mumia* or *vis vitalis*.

This is interesting because the German doctor Anton Mesmer who rediscovered this energy later, never bothered about plants and thought the energy was contained only in animals and humans.

Paracelsus, probably because he had understood that life is energy, and that all our dysfunctions in the body, as Chinese medicine knows since millennia, are obstructions of the vital energy flow, or *emotional flow*, was a phenomenally successful healer.

Yet because of his tempestuous character and his pride, he had to struggle hard against jealousy and also against the Church-driven authorities who reproached him he was doing black magic.

He had to stand trial for this cause, but he won the trial and was released. The social reject that was going along with his persecution was not too hard for him to bear as he was a *wandering scholar* and healer for long periods in his life, thus traveling around.

ALTERNATIVE MEDICINE AND WELLNESS TECHNIQUES

From this knowledge that is to be found also in Chinese plant medicine, he lectured that certain plants are collateral for healing and certain others not. He proposed to take only the *essences* from these plants, as this was later done by Samuel Hahnemann and Edward Bach in homeopathy, and to distill them as tinctures in which their energetic codes harmoniously melt into a higher form of unison vibration.

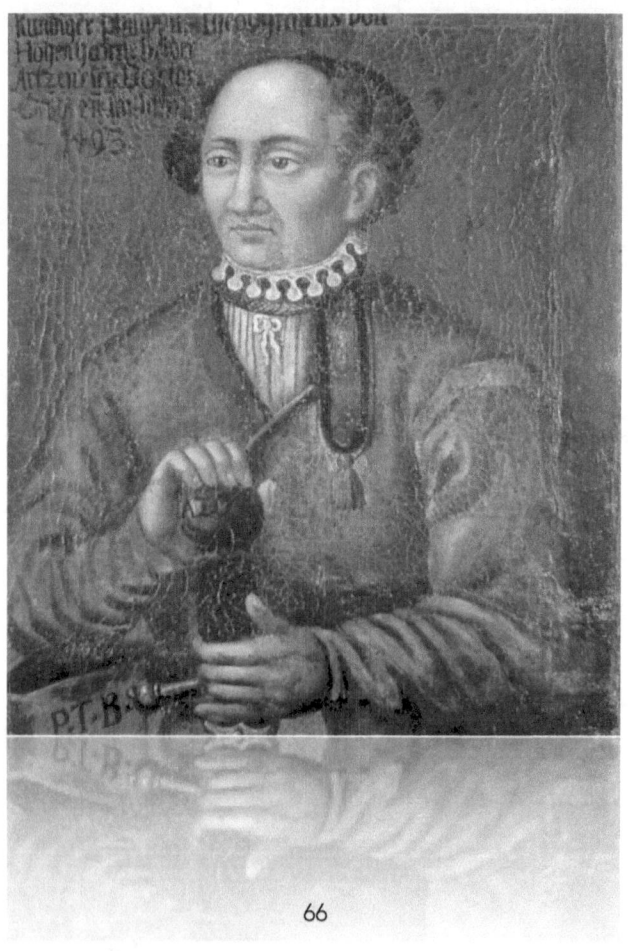

HOMEOPATHY

Here are some quotes from Manly P. Hall's book *The Secret Teachings of All Ages (1928/2003)* about Paracelsus that I find so pertinent that I would like to reproduce them here. In chapter XXIV, and the first sub-chapter, entitled *The Paracelsian System of Medical Philosophy*, Manly P. Hall writes:

> Paracelsus felt that the healing of the sick was of far greater importance than the maintaining of an orthodox medical standing, so he sacrificed what might otherwise have been a dignified medical career and at the cost of lifelong persecution bitterly attacked the therapeutic systems of his day. He was a true explorer of Nature's arcanum. Many authorities have held the opinion that he was the discoverer of mesmerism, and that Mesmer evolved the art as the result of studying the writings of this great Swiss physician. The utter contempt which Paracelsus felt for the narrow systems of medicine in vogue during his lifetime, and his conviction of their inadequacy, are best expressed in his own quaint way: 'But the number of diseases that originate from some unknown causes are far greater than those that come from mechanical causes, and for such diseases our physicians know no cure because not knowing such causes they cannot remove them.' (Id., 345)
>
> There is one vital substance in nature upon which all things subsist. It is called archaeus, or vital life force, and is synonymous with the astral light or spiritual air of the ancients. This vital energy has its origin in the spiritual body of the earth. Every created thing has two bodies, one visible and substantial, the other invisible

and transcendent. The latter consists of an ethereal counterpart of the physical form; it constitutes the vehicle of archaeus, and may be called the vital body. This etheric shadow sheath is not dissipated by death, but remains until the physical form is entirely disintegrated. It is derangements of this astral light body that cause much disease. (Id., 346)

Paracelsus, recognizing derangements of the etheric double as the most important cause of disease, sought to reharmonize its substances by bringing into contact with it other bodies whose vital energy could supply elements needed, or were strong enough to overcome the diseased conditions existing in the aura of the sufferer. Its invisible cause having been thus removed, the ailment speedily vanished. The vehicle for the archaeus, or vital life force, Paracelsus called the mumia. A good example of a physical mumia is vaccine, which is the vehicle of a semi-astral virus. Anything which serves as a medium for the transmission of the archaeus, whether it be organic or inorganic, truly physical or partly spiritualized, was termed a mumia. The most universal form of mumia was ether, which modern science has accepted as a hypothetical substance serving as a medium between the realm of vital energy and that of organic and inorganic substance. (Id., 347)

Paracelsus discovered that in many cases plants revealed by their shape the particular organs of the human body which they served most effectively. The medical system of Paracelsus was based on the theory that by removing the diseased etheric mumia from the organism of the patient and causing it to be accepted into the nature of some distant and disinterested thing of comparatively little value, it was possible to divert from the patient the flow of the archaeus which had been continually revitalizing and nourishing the malady. Its vehicle of expression being transplanted, the archaeus necessarily accompanied its mumia, and the patient recovered. (Id.)

Paracelsus' oeuvre is prolific both in quantity of content and scientific penetration. There are more than two hundred volumes of his writings still preserved, some hundred eighty of which are separately published editions before 1800. This remarkable collection appears to have been amassed carefully over a period of twenty or so years, commencing with Ferguson's first essay in Paracelsian research; a paper to the University Dialectic Society in 1873, entitled simply, *Paracelsus*, and culminating in the purchase of the extensive *Paralcelsia* belonging to Dr. Eduard Schubert sometime in 1894.

Schubert, with his friend Karl Sudhoff, had been interested in Paracelsus since his student days, and together they published *Paracelsus-Forschungen* between 1887 and 1889. They had also collaborated on a comprehensive bibliography of Paracelsus editions.

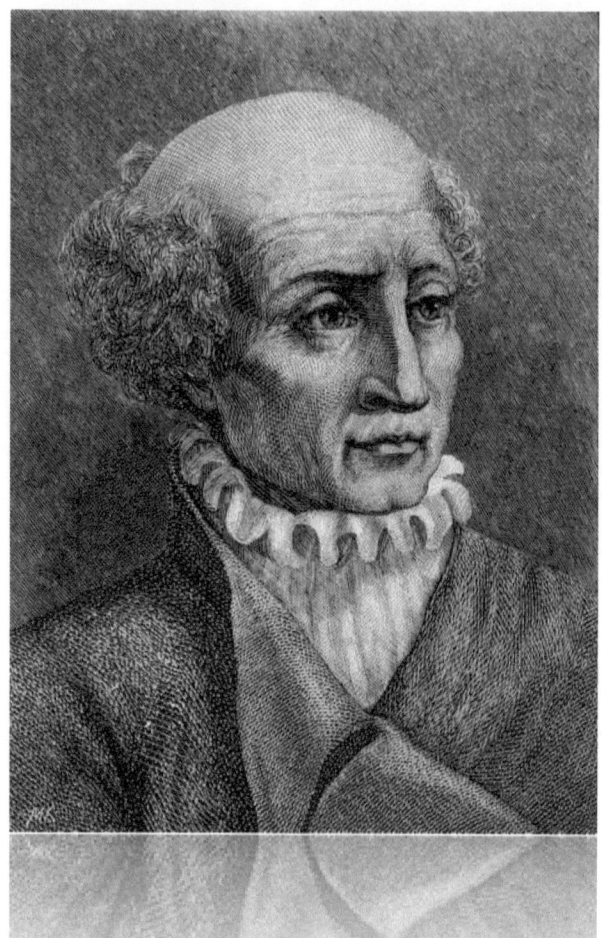

This was subsequently completed by Sudhoff, and finally published in 1894, two years after Schubert's death at the age of seventy. In the introduction to his *Bibliographia Paracelsia* Sudhoff lists the numerous libraries that he has used in the compilation of this monumental work.

SAMUEL HAHNEMANN

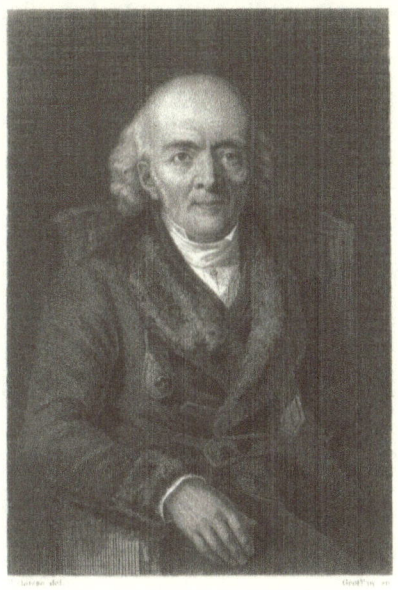

SAMUEL HAHNEMANN.

I find it amazing how Hahnemann discovered the basic principles of homeopathy he, a traditional physician with an antipathy against medicine because he, just like Paracelsus before him, was appalled at the blunt ignorance of Western medicine and the subtle and sometimes brutal treatments it bestowed upon the patient as the suffering agent. And just like Paracelsus, Hahnemann became aware that traditional medicine was just treating the symptoms of diseases and had no idea of the underlying causes because it ignored a holistic and comprehensive concept of *health*. Thus, Hahnemann began to systematically test substances for the effect they produced on a healthy individual and tried to deduce from this the ills they would heal. And he discovered that these dilutions, when done according to his technique of *succussion,* that is, the systematic mixing through vigorous shaking, and *potentization*, were effective in producing symptoms. Thus, instead of directly jumping to curing symptoms, he was first producing those symptoms with substances—and the surprising discovery he made was that typically the substance that was producing the symptom was the one that was curing the disease.

Hahnemann began practicing medicine again using his new technique, which soon attracted other doctors. He first published an article about the homeopathic approach to medicine in a German medical journal in 1796; in 1810, he wrote his *Organon of the Medical Art*, the first systematic treatise on the subject. Let me give you a preview of this oeuvre, which is published entirely on the Internet.

HOMEOPATHY

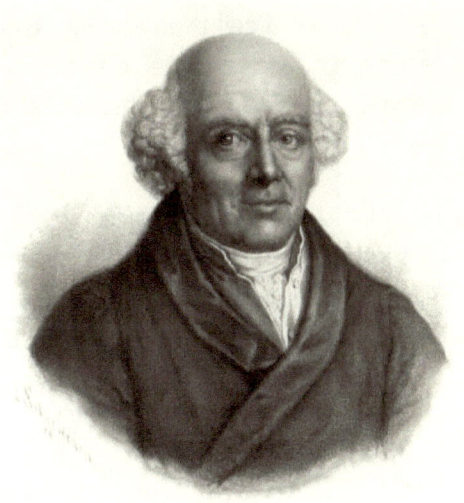

Samuel Hahnemann

§1 The physician's high and only mission is to restore the sick to health, to cure, as it is termed. His mission is not, however, to construct so-called systems, by interweaving empty speculations and hypotheses concerning the internal essential nature of the vital processes and the mode in which diseases originate in the interior of the organism, (whereon so many physicians have hitherto ambitiously wasted their talents and their time); nor is it to attempt to give countless explanations regarding the phenomena in diseases and their proximate cause (which must ever remain concealed), wrapped in unintelligible words and an inflated abstract mode of expression, which should sound very learned in order to astonish the ignorant—whilst sick humanity sighs in vain for aid. Of such learned reveries (to which the name of theoretic medicine is given, and for which special professorships are instituted) we have had quite enough, and it is now high time that all who call themselves physicians should at length cease to deceive suffering mankind with mere talk, and begin now, instead, for once to act, that is, really to help and to cure.

§2 The highest ideal of cure is rapid, gentle and permanent restoration of the health, or removal and annihilation of the disease in its whole extent, in the shortest, most reliable, and most harmless way, on easily comprehensible principles.

§3 If the physician clearly perceives what is to be cured in diseases, that is to say, in every individual case of disease (knowledge of disease, indication), if he clearly perceives what is curative in medicines, that is to say, in each individual medicine (knowledge of medical powers), and if he knows how to adapt, according to clearly defined principles, what is curative in medicines to what he has discovered to be undoubtedly morbid in the patient, so that the recovery must ensue—to adapt it, as well in respect to the suitability of the medicine most appropriate according to its mode of action to the case before him (choice of the remedy, the medicine indicated), as also in respect to the exact mode of preparation and quantity of it required (proper dose), and the proper period for repeating the dose;—if, finally, he knows the obstacles to recovery in each case and is aware how to remove them, so that the restoration may be permanent, then he understands how to treat judiciously and rationally, and he is a true practitioner of the healing art.

§4 He is likewise a preserver of health if he knows the things that derange health and cause disease, and how to remove them from persons in health.

HOMEOPATHY

§5 Useful to the physician in assisting him to cure are the particulars of the most probable exciting cause of the acute disease, as also the most significant points in the whole history of the chronic disease, to enable him to discover its fundamental cause, which is generally due to a chronic miasm. In these investigations, the ascertainable physical constitution of the patient (especially when the disease is chronic), his moral and intellectual character, his occupation, mode of living and habits, his social and domestic relations, his age, sexual function, etc., are to be taken into consideration.

§6 The unprejudiced observer—well aware of the futility of transcendental speculations which can receive no confirmation from experience—be his powers of penetration ever so great, takes note of nothing in every individual disease, except the changes in the health of the body and of the mind (morbid phenomena, accidents, symptoms) which can be perceived externally by means of the senses; that is to say, he notices only the deviations from the former healthy state of the now diseased individual, which are felt by the patient himself, remarked by those around him and observed by the physician. All these perceptible signs represent the disease in its whole extent, that is, together they form the true and only conceivable portrait of the disease.

Edward Bach

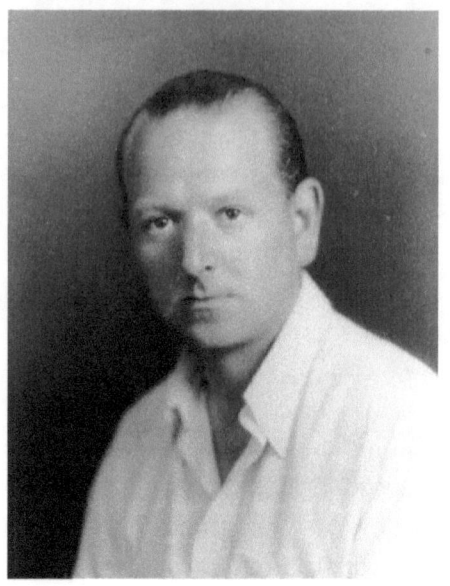

Dr. Edward Bach (1886–1936) has contributed in a unique and outstanding way to homeopathy and generally, to natural healing.

I came in touch with his flower remedies in 1997 when, returning from a two-year business trip from Asia to Germany, I was facing a dangerously low condition of vital energy due to a prolonged intake of antibiotics given from traditional doctors in order to fight recurring diarrhea. From the natural healer I went to see, I learnt that the *therapeutic value* of Bach essences lies not in curing the physical symptoms of illness but in addressing the emotional state of the

HOMEOPATHY

sufferer, wherein lie the roots of illness. For this reason the application, I heard, of these 38 simple, natural essences spans the gamut, not only of human ailments, but also illnesses of other living beings. An emotional state, unlike an illness, crosses boundaries of species and illness type.

The most interesting in this kind of therapy was how the healer found the essence that was resonating with my illness. The female practitioner who had studied hypnosis and Reiki with a powerful Filipino spiritual healer, explained me very patiently the various methods for finding the energy essence corresponding to my own organism's energy code and asked me which one I preferred.

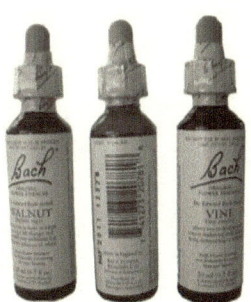

I chose the most direct method, hypnosis, and the experience was going to be a particularly revealing one for me. She was sitting at a forty-five degree angle at my right and asked me to put my left hand in her right hand. Then she told me to look in her eyes while she would take one flacon after the other in her left hand to sense the effect the vibration of the plant essence had on my organism.

Never before was I hypnotized so easily, so effectively and so joyfully. It was a very agreeable condition and I felt very clearly how each of the essences impacted energetically upon me.

The healer said I was going to feel either joyful, peaceful, positive and happy, which indicated that the essence was right for me, or I was feeling queer, anxious and negative, which was indicating that the essence was not compatible with my aura's vibrational structure.

This was how I was going to choose one of the plant remedies. The treatment was the most effective one can imagine. It was almost miraculous. I was completely cured within three months, and with only six sessions.

By the time he died in 1936, Dr. Bach had discovered the 38 remedies that were needed to treat every possible emotional state, with each individual remedy being aimed at a particular emotion or characteristic. Sometimes people find it strange that only 38 can deal with everything, but in fact used in combination, over 292 million different mental states are covered.

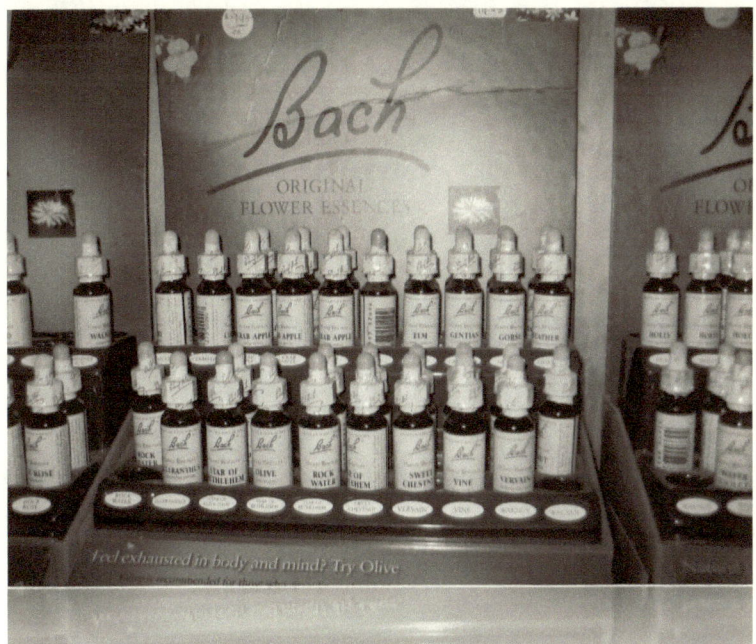

Within the Bach flower system, and among the 38 essences, there are twelve plants that Bach himself called *The Twelve Healers*, which are of particular importance. I will briefly mention them below and describe them one by one. It is all about vibration we are talking when we talk about flower remedies. The universe is a vibrational cosmos with no finite particles, but dynamic energy patterns. Every flower has a unique energy pattern. There are energy frequencies that are particular to Agrimony, for example, and other energy frequencies that are characteristic for Gentian. While perennial science since millennia understood that life is basically vibration, this is a relatively new insight for Western science, and it is now first of all quantum physics, and second, systems theory, that bring the evidence long needed to integrate vibrational healing into the Western medical system.

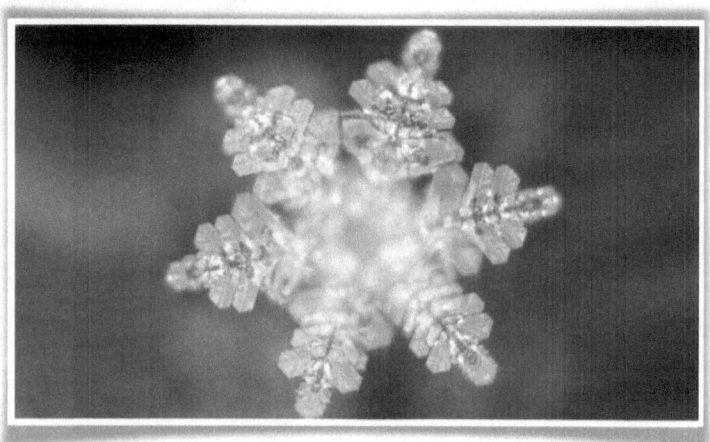

Water research has shown that flowers can cause water to vibrate with a different sort of energy. This means that the essence of the flower has a vibration that is imprinted upon the water in which it is placed. The water, being made up of vibrational energy itself, retains some of the vibration of the flower that was soaked in it.

HOMEOPATHY

Masaru Emoto claims that water has a memory, which means that the flower's etheric imprint is stored in the water, and can actually be transferred from the water at a later time to other objects (or beings) also made of vibrational energy.

My research on emotions showed that all emotions have a particular energy—love, despair, anger, fear, revolt—one can consider each of these as a different vibrational pattern.

Dr. Bach considered negative energetic states, negative emotions, to be the source of disease in the body, a theory supported by other natural healers. Dr. Bach also thought that these energetic states can be transformed, and that one of the transformational methods he discovered was the use of the *vibrational patters* of flowers—it was then that *Flower Essence Therapy* was born.

Through basically a method of trial and error, Dr. Bach developed a system of therapy using the vibrational patterns of flowers, imprinted into spring water, to transform the emotional patters of human beings. He showed through numerous case studies that plant essences, properly selected and applied, can be effective in treating the negative energies which underlie most disease states. Further, flower essences can be used to assist in transforming any negative emotional state, be it temporary and transitive, or a more ingrained long-term pattern.

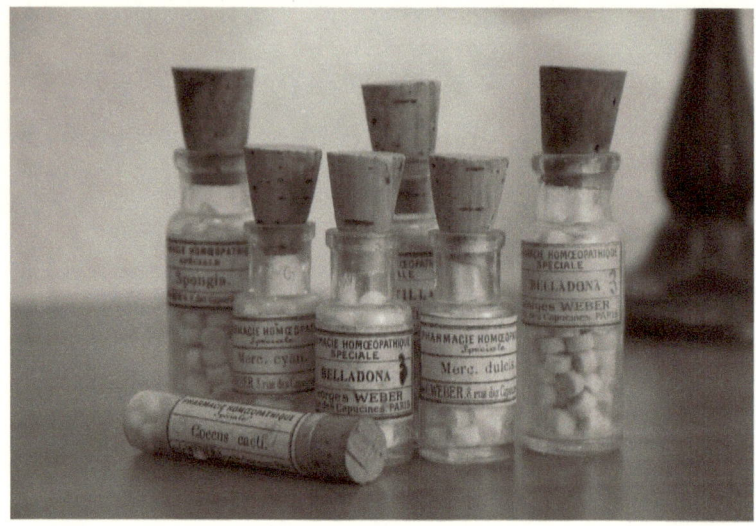

Dr. Bach then categorized the original 38 flower essences into 3 categories to assist in their application. The categories are the *12 Healers* which reflect and transform our essential nature, the *7 Helpers* to assist with chronic conditions, and the *Second 19* that relate to more immediate traumas or difficulties. The 12 Healers were designated by Dr. Bach as the flower essences that help the individual transform the source of discord at the very core of their being.

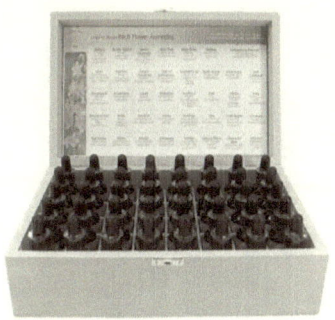

These twelve essences are meant to address the twelve archetypal groups of humanity; the twelve primary personalities as Dr. Bach saw them. Some have gone so far as to relate these to the twelve signs of the Zodiac, though it is unclear as to whether this relationship was drawn by Dr. Bach himself. These twelve essences are an excellent starting point for any journey into flower essence healing, as it is often times our root disharmony or karmic imbalance that is the source of many ailments in our lives.

ALTERNATIVE MEDICINE AND WELLNESS TECHNIQUES

Masaru Emoto

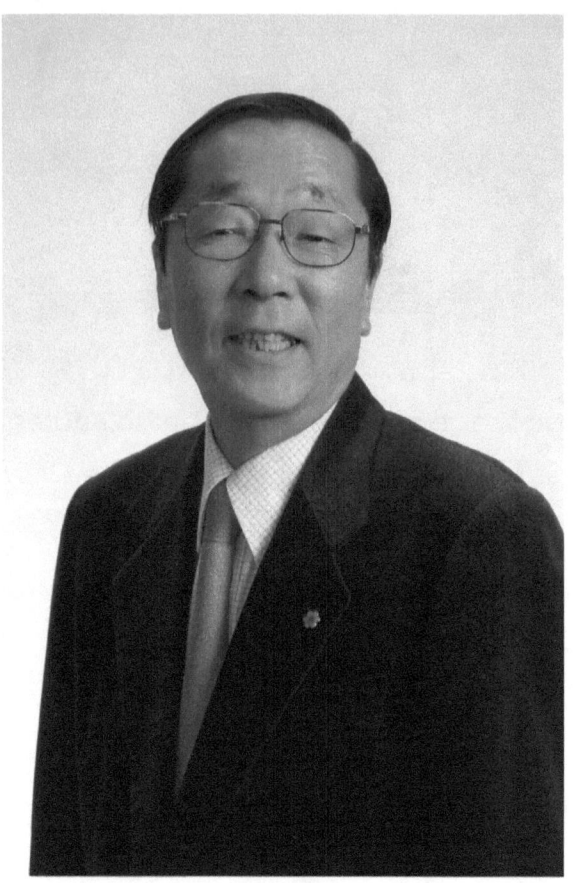

Dr. Masaru Emoto, Doctor of Alternative Medicine at the Open International University, Japan, and President of I.H.M. General Research Institute, became world-famous through the spectacular movie *'What the Bleep Do We Know' (2005)* and it was through this film that I got to know about his outstanding research on the memory of water.

HOMEOPATHY

When Dr. Emoto's books *The Hidden Messages in Water (2004)* and *The Secret Life of Water (2005)* reached me, they reached me right in time, at a moment when I had caught Dengue fever. But not only because I was in considerable distress being treated in a quite murky, unhealthy, inattentive and dirty Chinese hospital, the more significant thing about it all is the date. The day the books arrived, was the 25th of July.

Dr. Emoto reports in *The Secret Life of Water* that according to the Mayan Calendar, the new year starts on July 26, and the day before was called 'the day out of time.' When you divide 365 by 28, you get 13 months and one extra day. This day was a celebration day during which prayers were offered. And what I did that evening was to pray, with all my soul, and putting stickers with the words LOVE AND GRATITUDE on bottles with mineral water; in fact, I spent the whole evening reading *The Hidden Messages in Water*.

As the serum treatment and injections I got in the hospital and the morning and the strong antibiotic pills I got for the afternoon rendered me very weak, tired, extremely sweaty and dizzy, I drank a lot of water and, following the advice of the doctor, was eating only rice porridge with fish.

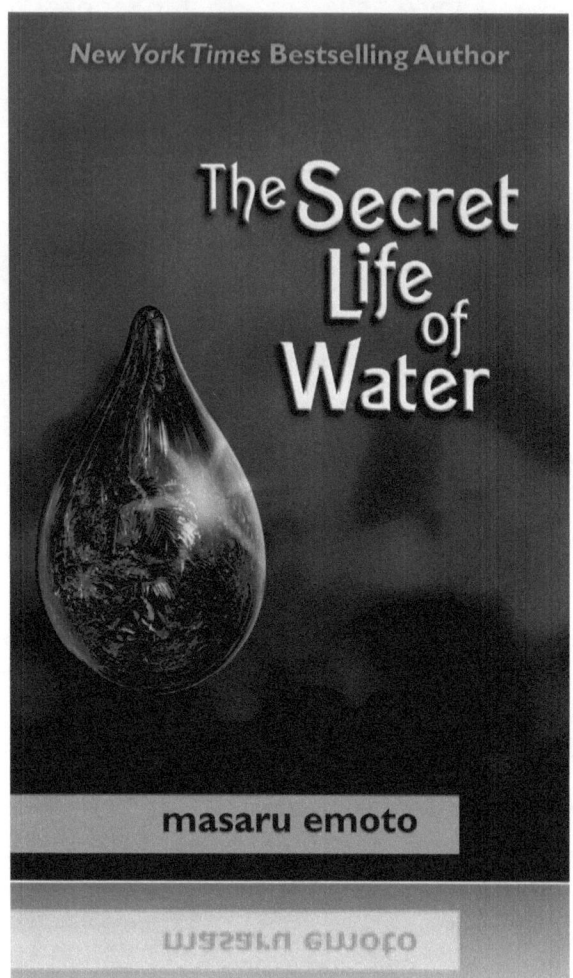

However, that evening was a silent prayer for the water inside of my body and indeed, the next morning I felt significantly better and for the first time, the fever was down. That was the morning of the 26th of July. And for me it was indeed a new year.

HOMEOPATHY

Dr. Emoto's voice, his *deep commitment* to the cause of a tortured earth, humankind and waters in distress has deeply penetrated into my soul and finds a complete resonance with the whole of my being. And the next day I composed on the piano a little piece I entitled *Prayer to the Water*.

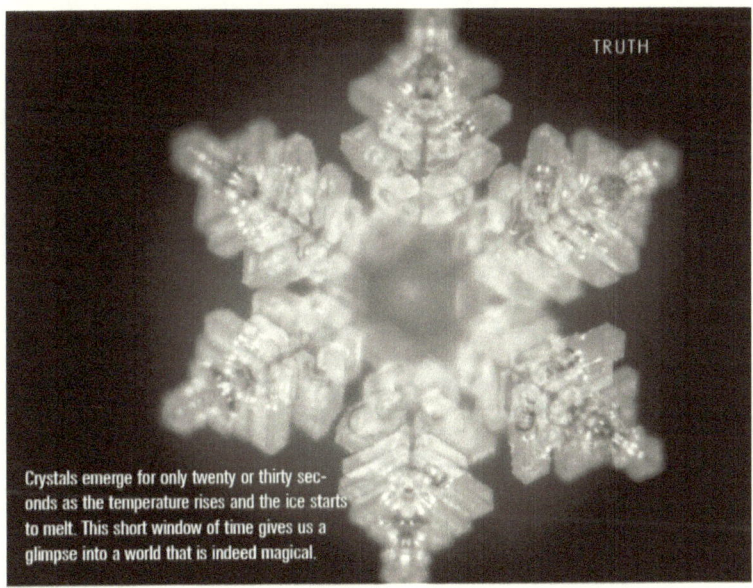

TRUTH

Crystals emerge for only twenty or thirty seconds as the temperature rises and the ice starts to melt. This short window of time gives us a glimpse into a world that is indeed magical.

Without wanting to diminish Emoto's research in any way, I may want to mention that water research was not his invention.

Max Freedom Long became aware that the Kahunas used a handy metaphor for describing the *mana* force; they associated it with water as a liquid substance that represents the juice of life; from this basic idea, the Kahunas extrapolated the metaphor of the human being as a tree or plant, 'the roots being the low self, the trunk and branches the middle self, and the leaves the high self.' While the sap circulating through roots, branches and leaves vividly illustrated the nature of the mana force.

> — See Max Long, The Secret Science at Work: The Huna Method as a Way of Life (1995), 17.

The *Essenes*, the first Christians gnostics, interestingly had the same or a very similar imagery regarding the vital force. It was for this reason, as Edmond Bordeaux-Szekely found, that they had given so much importance to the water purification ritual.

They spoke of a *Goddess of the Water*, a vital force that they believed was inhabiting water and that was purifying us through the use of daily cold showers taken in free nature and with water that was taken directly from a lively source such as a mountain stream or age-old well that was known to contain highly pure water.

> — See Edmond Bordeaux-Szekely, *Gospel of the Essenes* (1988).

HOMEOPATHY

Now, the amazing research done with water and vibrations by Masaru Emoto fully confirms these findings with new and surprising evidence.

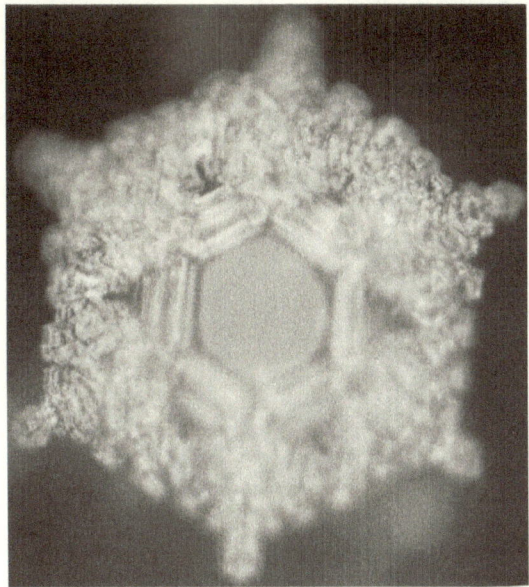
Love and Gratitude

Dr. Emoto found the enormous implications of vibration by looking at the vibrational code of water that he calls *hado*. In the Japanese spiritual tradition, *hado* is indeed considered as a vibrational code that, similar to *ki*, the life energy, has healing properties and transformative powers. Literally translated, *hado* means wave motion or vibration. Once we are aware of it in our everyday lives, Emoto showed, *hado* can spark great changes in our physical space and emotional wellbeing. What Emoto teaches can thus be called hado awareness or *vibrational awareness*, as part of a general acute awareness of how we influence our environment, and our lives, through our thoughts and emotions. The point of departure is thus to recognize and acknowledge that in every thought and emotion, a specific vibration manifests.

It is interesting that in *Feng Shui*, only flowing water is considered to contain the positive *ch'i* energy, while stagnant water is deemed to contain a rather harmful and retrograde variant of *ch'i* which is called *sha*.

> —See, for example, Ong Hean-Tatt, Amazing Scientific Basis of Feng Shui (1997), Karen Kingston, Creating Sacred Space with Feng Shui (1997), Lillian Too, Feng Shui (1994), Man-Ho Kwok, The Feng Shui Kit (1995), Nancilee Wydra, Feng Shui: The Book of Cures (1996), Richard Craze, Feng Shui Book and Card Pack (1997).

The next amazing discovery that Emoto came about was the fact that water has a memory—a memory far longer than our transient lifetimes. And third, that we can learn from water, by allowing it to resonate within us. Only a few researchers have confirmed this assumption until now, and one of them

HOMEOPATHY

is the reputed science philosopher Ervin Laszlo. He writes in his study *Science and the Akashic Field* (2004):

> Water has a remarkable capacity to register and conserve information, as indicated by, among other things, homeopathic remedies that remain effective even when not a single molecule of the original substance remains in a dilution.

— Ervin Laszlo, Science and the Akashic Field (2004), p. 53.

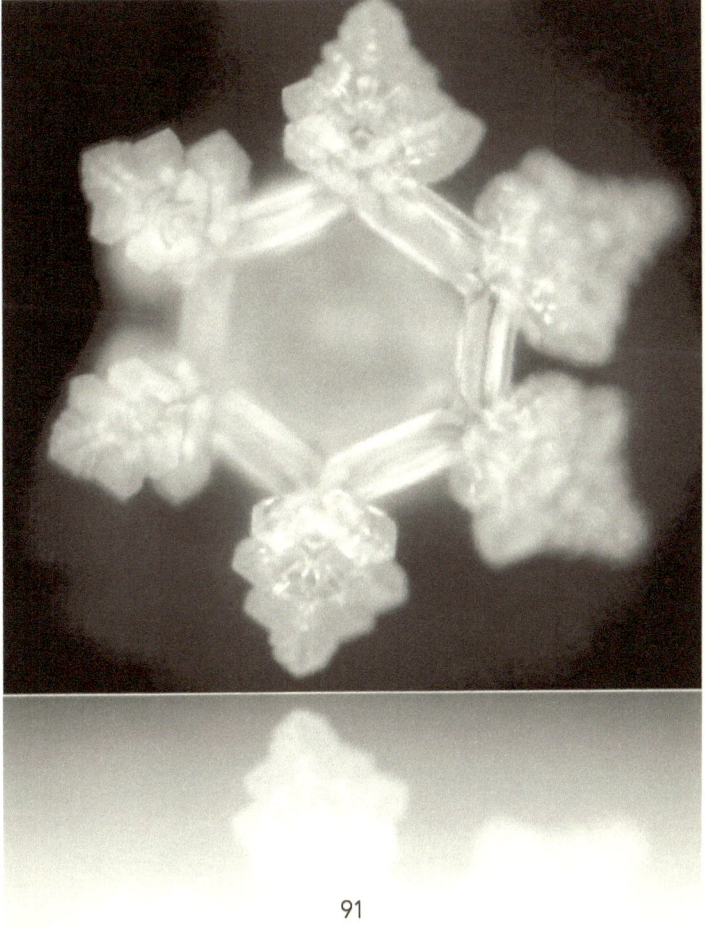

Kirlian Photography

The Final Evidence of the Luminous Energy Field

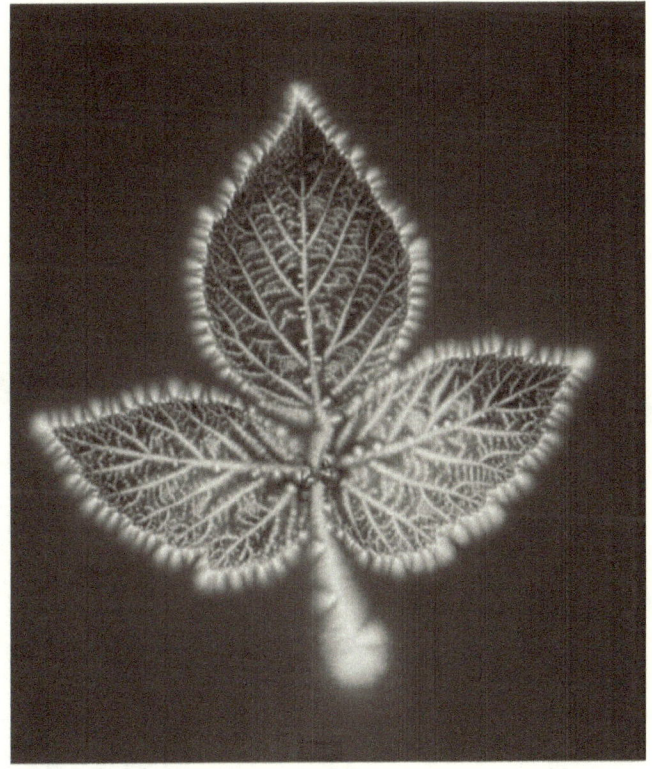

Kirlian Photography refers to a form of contact print photography, theoretically associated with high-voltage. It is named after Dr. Kirlian, who in 1939 discovered that if an object on a photographic plate is

ALTERNATIVE MEDICINE AND WELLNESS TECHNIQUES

subjected to a strong electric field, an image is created on the plate. Dr. Kirlian's work, that was first called *corona discharge photography* was explored by other researchers such as Lichtenberg and Tesla. Yet Kirlian took the development of the effect further than any of his predecessors.

Kirlian Photography is today credited with being the first attempt to successfully photograph the bioplasmatic *aura* or *energy field* around living beings, plants, animals and humans. The photographs show the aura as a colorful halo stretching a few inches around the physical body.

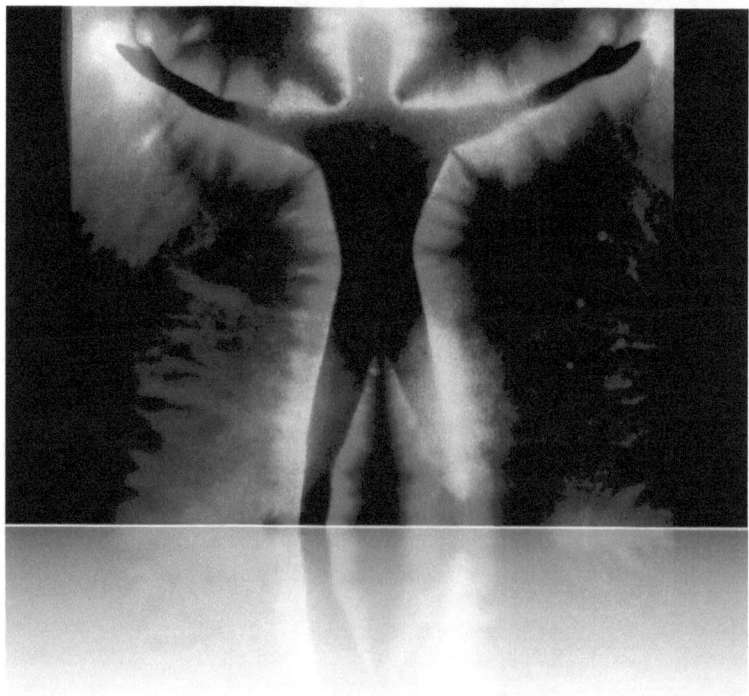

KIRLIAN PHOTOGRAPHY

One of the more striking aspects of Kirlian photography is its ability to illuminate the acupuncture points of the human body.

An experiment advanced as *evidence of energy fields* generated by living entities involves taking Kirlian contact photographs of a picked leaf at set periods, its gradual withering being said to correspond with a decline in the strength of the aura.

Another striking fact proven by Kirlian photography is that the aura bears the memory of the whole body even when a part of the body is lost. This was shown with cutting off a leaf from a branch. The Kirlian photo still shows the missing leaf, which gave rise to explaining the fact why war veterans can indeed suffer from post-amputation pain in their missing arms or legs, a fact that previously was always downplayed as paranoid or a product of vivid fantasy.

It was back in the 1980s that I heard for the first time about Kirlian Photography. I thought for myself that that *had to be invented* as since my school days I had been aware that Western science is blinding out the most essential, the cosmic life energy, the bioplasmatic energy that is both in the cell plasma and the aura. Kirlian photography was perhaps the first convincing evidence of this energy.

I also became aware that with so many great discoveries, including *Reich's Greatest Discoveries*, they have been made in the first decades of the 20th century but were ferociously aggressed by the science establishment at first, and until today are more or less blinded out from the mainstream Western scientific worldview. Many of these discoveries have been promoted by those, who like Wilhelm Reich, were defamed and labeled as quacks and charlatans, but who, as we know today, were simply scientific geniuses.

—See Peter Fritz Walter, Wilhelm Reich and the Function of the Orgasm (Great Minds Series, Vol. 11), 2015/2017.

It was at that time that I had my first ideas about creating a science that inquires into emotions and sexuality from the bioenergetic perspective and that I later called *Emonics*.

I was especially baffled by the fact that Kirlian Photography revealed the fact that memory is coded in the aura or the luminous body, which shows that *memory is actually a function of the luminous energy field*, not a matter of neurons and of mysterious substances in the brain.

Hence, memory is not located in the brain, and as this fact is in such flagrant contradiction with the myths of neurology and brain research, I was encouraged to research further on these lines.

There are several books among those I discussed in my book reviews that take reference to Kirlian Photography, one of them with more than a short reference. It is this book, which I reviewed and highly recommend:

Shafica Karagulla

The Chakras
With Dora van Gelder Kunz
Correlations between Medical Science and Clairvoyant Observation (1989)
Wheaton: Quest Books, 1989.

Kyudo

A Japanese Martial Art

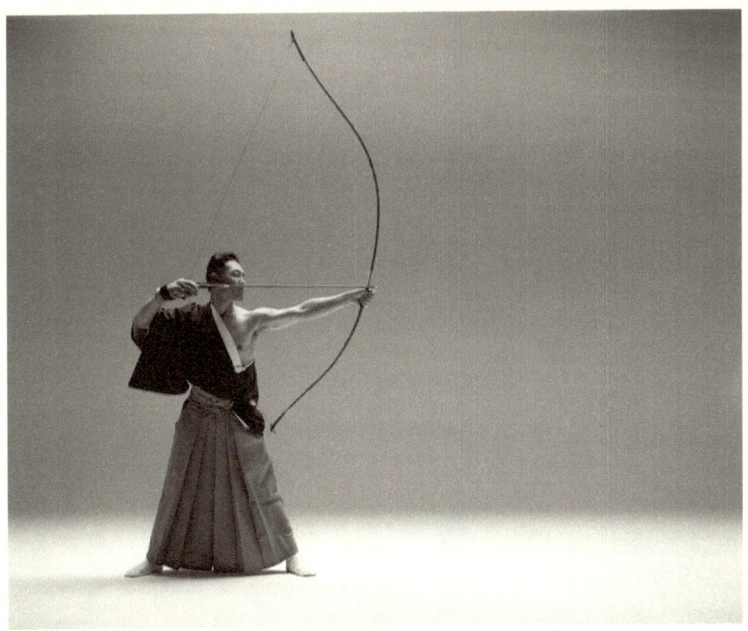

What is Kyudo?

Kyudo, literally meaning way of the bow, is the Japanese art of archery. It is a modern Japanese martial art *(gendai budo)*. It is estimated that there are approximately half a million practitioners of Kyudo today.

In Japan, by most accounts, the number of female Kyudo practitioners is at least equal to or greater than the number of male practitioners. In its purest form, Kyudo is practiced as an art and as a means of moral and spiritual development.

Kyudo in Germany

Many archers practice Kyudo as a sport, with marksmanship being paramount. However, the goal most devotees of Kyudo seek is correct shooting and correct hitting. When the spirit and balance of the shooting is correct the result will be for the arrow to arrive in the target, which is of course a metaphor for success in life at large.

Kyudo in Japan

To give oneself completely to the shooting is the spiritual goal. In this respect, many Kyudo practitioners believe that competition, examination, and any opportunity that places the archer in this uncompromising situation is important, while other practitioners will avoid competitions or examinations of any kind.

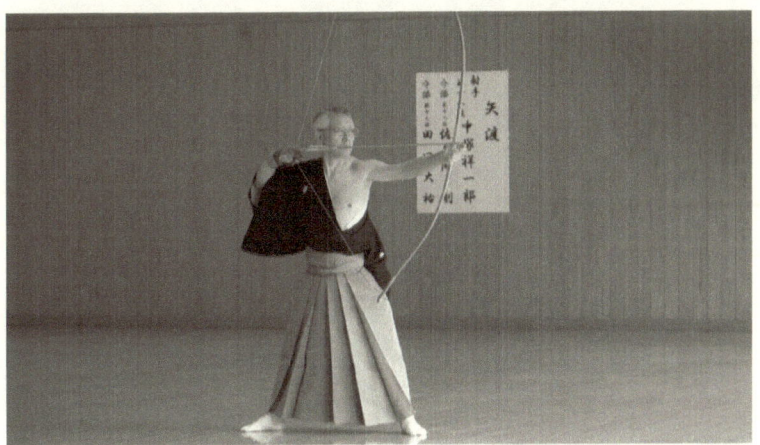

Naturopathy

An American Natural Healing System

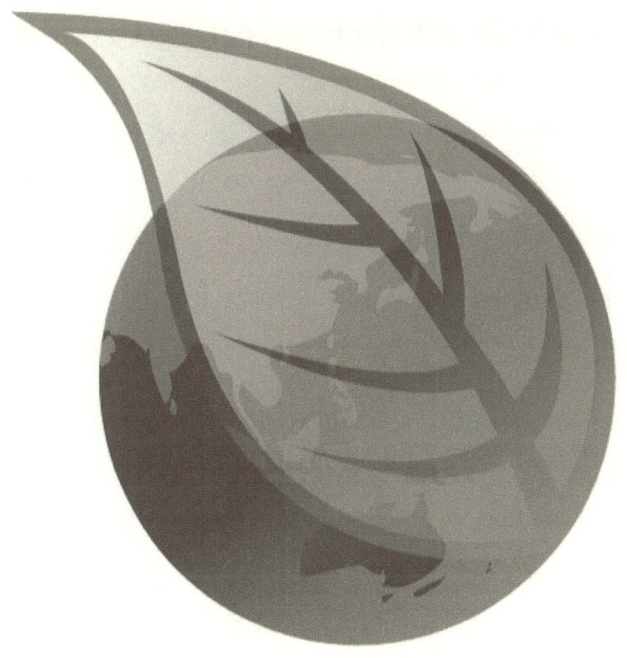

The Six Principles of Healing

1. Nature's Healing Power

2. Identify the Cause

3. Do No Harm

4. Whole Person Treatment

5. The Physician is Teacher

6. Disease Prevention

Nature's Healing Power

Using nature's inherent healing power implies to activate the body's self-healing ability, so that nature can exhibit its full healing power. Following this principle means the doctor should instruct the patient about getting enough sleep, doing some kind of exercise, feeding the body in natural ways and, if needed, considering a special diet, such as eating herbs, or algae, which as living organisms are antioxidants and contain the *essence of life*. Plants can gently move the body into health without side effects posed by some synthetic chemicals in modern pharmaceuticals.

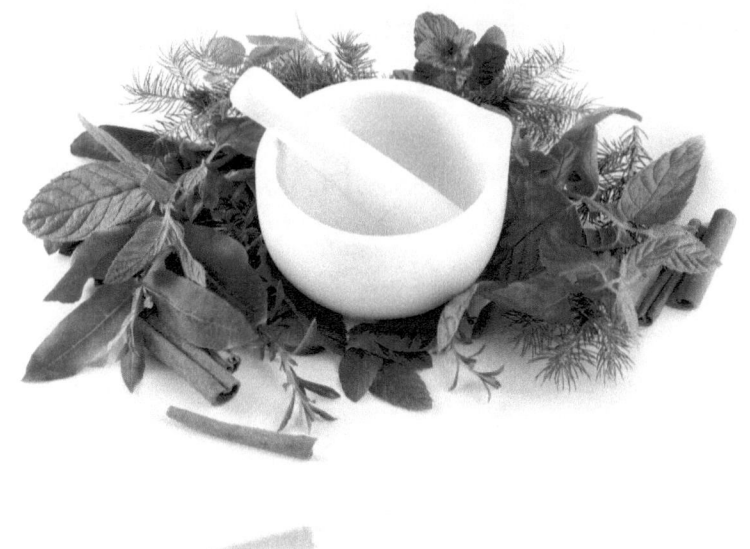

Identify the Cause

We have seen that Samuel Hahnemann strongly emphasized to find the root cause of the disease instead of speculating what the various symptoms may do or not do to the body.

It is logical that for healing to occur, the root cause of the disease must be found and eliminated. The cause of the disease may be located at various levels at once, the physical, mental, emotional, and spiritual levels. It is the naturopathic doctor's ostensible role to identify this root cause, in addition to alleviating suffering by treating symptoms.

Do No Harm

We have seen that Paracelsus was strongly motivated to become a natural healer because he saw the great harm doctors did to their patients at that time. This principle is perhaps the most important for natural healing in general, and for naturopathy, in particular. It goes without saying that the treatment of the disease should never do greater harm than the disease itself.

Whole Person Treatment

It goes without saying that an approach that targets the root cause of the disease, instead of curing the symptoms, is one that approaches the whole human, and eventually heals the whole human —not just body parts. That means treating the entire body, as well as the spiritual being within the physical person.

The Physician is Teacher

It is the role of the naturopath to educate the patient in naturopathic practice and encourage him or her to take responsibility for their health and wellbeing. This cooperative relationship between doctor and patient is essential to healing, while in modern medicine it is often neglected and replaced by applying machinery to the body 'machine' of the patient.

Disease Prevention

The ultimate goal of the naturopathic physician is prevention. The emphasis is on building health, not fighting illness. This is done by fostering healthy lifestyles, healthy beliefs, and healthy relationships.

OSTEOPATHY

The Eight Principles of Osteopathic Healing

What is Osteopathy?

Osteopathy is a uniquely American natural health care system that was developed about one hundred twenty years ago.

With a strong emphasis on the inter-relationship of the body's nerves, muscles, bones and organs, osteopaths apply the philosophy of treating the whole person.

Osteopathy is thus a holistic approach to healing, which includes prevention, diagnosis and treatment of illness, disease and injury using manual and physical therapies (OMM).

For non-American natural healers it may be difficult to understand the difference between osteopathy and naturopathy. It has been for me. In fact, there is no difference in principle but well one in applying the principle in practice. They are two different systems of health care, both of which are holistic and both of which do no harm to the patient

Osteopathic medicine is practiced by osteopathic physicians in the United States. Osteopaths educated in countries outside the U.S. are referred to by American osteopathic physicians as 'non-physician osteopaths.' Their scope of practice is limited largely to musculoskeletal conditions and treatment of some other conditions using manual treatment (OMM), not unlike chiropractors (although the distinction between the two professions remains important to both).

The Eight Principles of Osteopathy

These are the eight major principles of osteopathy and are widely accepted throughout the osteopathic community. They are taken from the curriculum of the *Kirksville College of Osteopathic Medicine*:

(1) The body is a unit.

(2) Structure and function are reciprocally inter-related.

(3) The body possesses self-regulatory mechanisms.

(4) The body has the inherent capacity to defend and repair itself.

(5) When the normal adaptability is disrupted, or when environmental changes overcome the body's capacity for self maintenance, disease may ensue.

(6) The movement of body fluids is essential to the maintenance of health.

(7) The nerves play a crucial part in controlling the fluids of the body.

(8) There are somatic components to disease that are not only manifestations of disease, but also are factors that contribute to the maintenance of the disease state.

These principles are not held by osteopaths to be empirical laws, nor contradictions to orthodox medical principles; they are thought to be the underpinnings of the osteopathic perspective on health and disease.

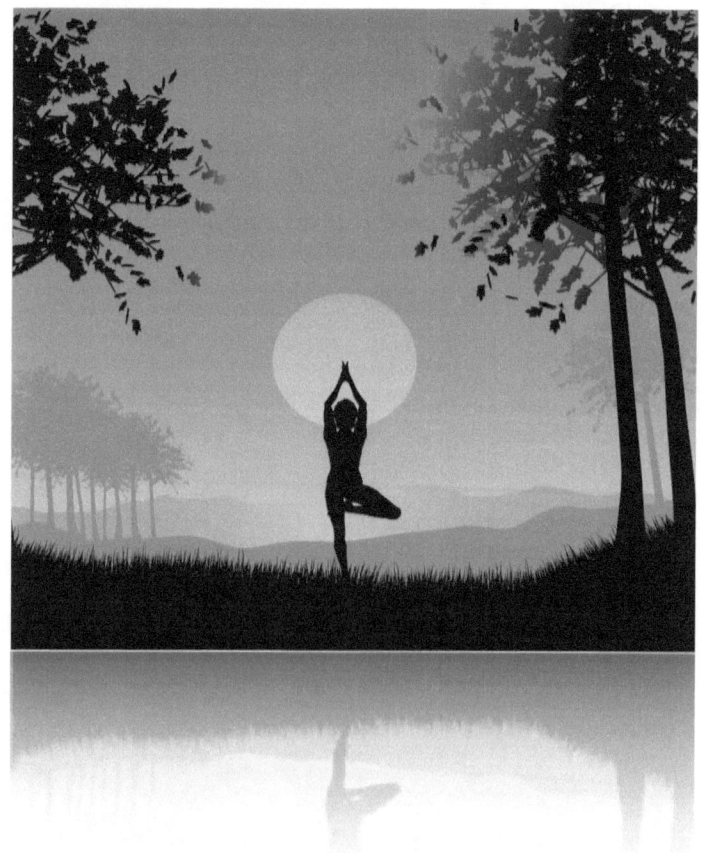

Qigong

The Art of Breathing

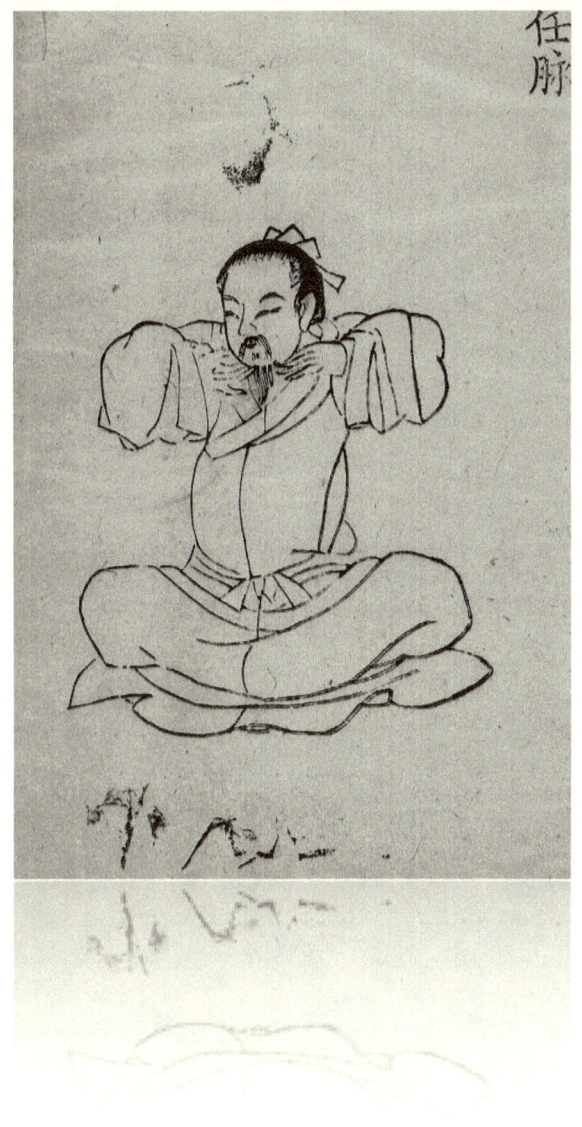

ALTERNATIVE MEDICINE AND WELLNESS TECHNIQUES

What is Qigong?

Qigong or *ch'i kung* refers to a wide variety of traditional cultivation practices that involve methods of accumulating, circulating, and working with the vital energy flow *(ch'i)* mainly through breathing and other body energy work.

Qigong is practiced for health maintenance purposes, as a therapeutic intervention, as a medical profession, a spiritual path and/or component of Chinese martial arts. The *ch'i* or *qi* means 'air' in Chinese, and, by extension, *life force*, dynamic energy or cosmic breath.

Gong means work applied to a discipline or the resultant level of skill; qigong is thus breath work or energy work.

Wikipedia

Most Western medical practitioners and many practitioners of traditional Chinese medicine, as well as the Chinese government, view qigong as a set of breathing and movement exercises, with possible benefits to health through stress reduction and exercise. Others see qigong in more metaphysical terms, claiming that qi can be circulated through channels called meridians.

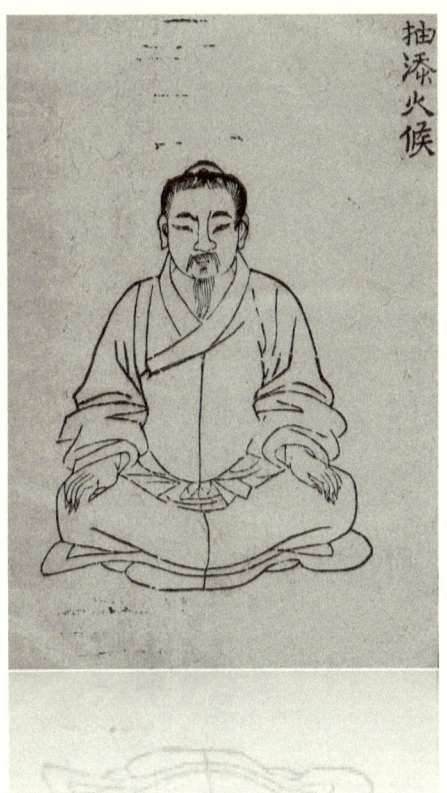

The Qigong Posture

Qigong is a Chinese system of breath control and physical postures that support right breathing. Right breathing activates the flow of the *ch'i* or vital energy in the organism and thereby helps prevent disease. It also helps accelerating healing processes.

I have practiced Qigong over years and can testify that it purifies our inner energy channels, and contributes to health and mental clarity. It also helps to balance our emotions.

When practicing Qigong, one should ideally be on a healthy diet, avoid alcoholic beverages, avoid smoking and eat lots of fresh food, salads, sprouts, beans and fibers. One should also avoid meat and dairy products.

Qigong for Healing Sexual Sadism

For people who suffer from a sadistic affliction, or recurrent rape desires, I recommend Qigong, among other self-awareness techniques, as I have elaborated them in various publications. In fact, these desires, so much blamed in Western society as a sort of 'moral decadence' have nothing 'moral' to them, nor anything 'immoral.' They are, functionally speaking, energy stray patterns, that is, a result of the vital energy being blocked in certain areas of the body—especially the areas of the chest and neck, the genital area and the area between the anus and the testicles, as well as the 'hara' point, the underbelly. Those armored areas in the body block the flow of the ch'i, thereby creating inner tension; and it is precisely this tension that induces the desire to rape for unconsciously this desire is actually a desire to get rid of the tension.

Thus, from a functional point of view the man who desires to rape, desires in reality to get into a healthy streaming of his vital energy; and while he may be steeped in daydreaming about raping this or the other sexual object, what he *really* wishes is to be healthy again, and get rid of the surplus tension of his vital organism.

It goes without saying that when we are caught in moralism, we cannot think functionally and thus cannot understand the dynamics of rape. We are then also not able to heal the affliction, for that's what it is, a pathological state of the sexual energy.

Wilhelm Reich (1897-1957) was the first medical doctor and psychoanalyst who has explained rape and other sexual dysfunctions from a functional perspective, declaring our age-old moralistic tradition a fallacy.

He was not understood at his lifetime, and even slandered and declared a quack, yet today, and with the additional knowledge of Traditional Chinese Medicine and Qigong, as a practice, we know that he was right in that the rape affliction can be healed through Qigong techniques.

Qigong clarifies and clears strayed energy patterns in our human aura, and brings them back into the unified energy field, so that sexual attraction is again tender, warm, with hot melting emotions and streaming sensations in the body, instead of the cold and violent urge for quick and sometimes brutal abreaction that characterizes the sadistic affliction.

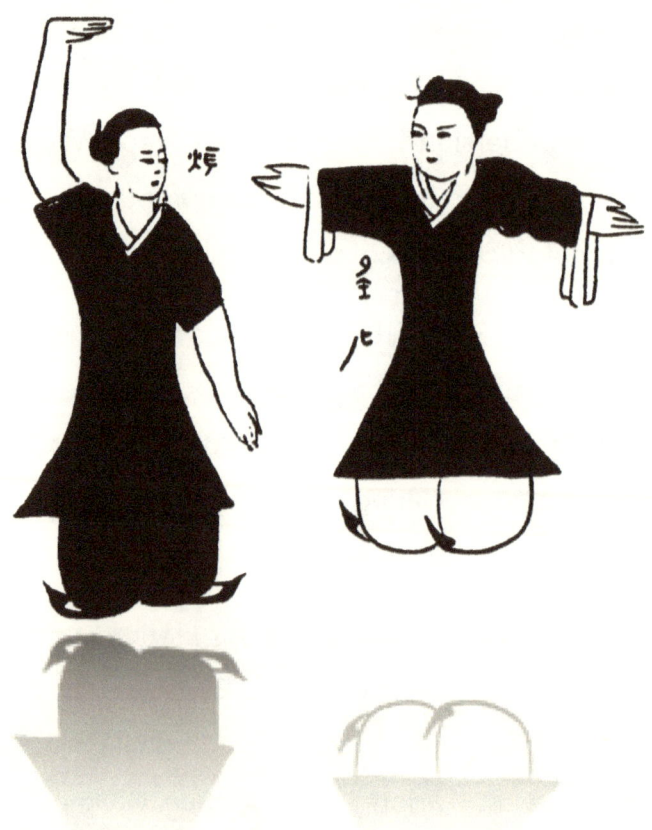

Radionics

The Unknown Medical Science

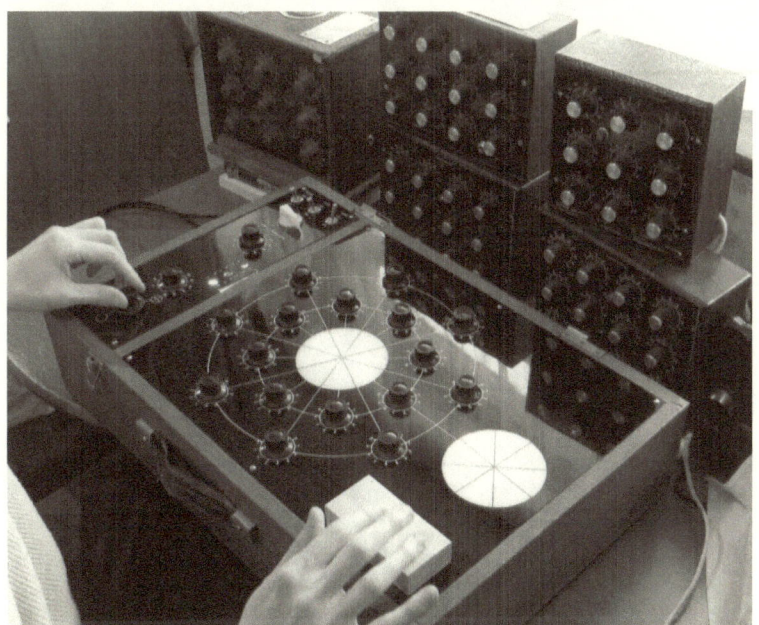

What is Radionics?

Radionics is a science that to this day is understood only by a small elite of scientists, as it is so far still largely located within the gray area between official science and spirituality, out of the shot lines of the great public. But that does not diminish its importance. It owns its existence to two *rather distinct* streams of influence, for one the esoteric spiritual teachings of Alice Bailey, on one hand, and the experimental findings of the Russian-French scientist Georges Lakhovsky (1869–1942), on the other.

To explain the complex technique of this science in simple words, let me describe Radionics as a healing technique that uses insights into the laws of cell vibration for the purpose of curing disease.

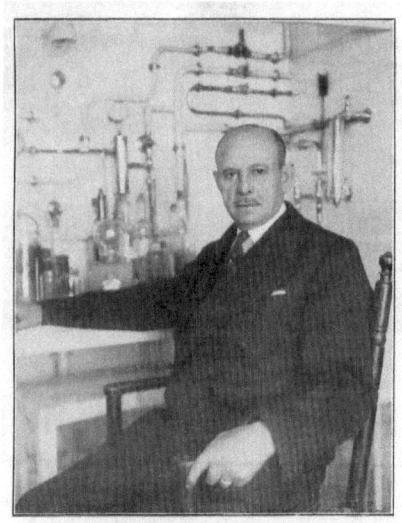

GEORGES LAKHOVSKY

Radionics has been compared with Wilhelm Reich's *orgonomy*, with the laying-on of hands and with spiritual healing, but matters are more complex than that. An in-depth study of this complex science would be needed to really explain its functioning.

I have reviewed George Lakhovsky's major writings, among them *The Secret of Life (1929)*.

Lakhovsky found that all living cells possess attributes that normally are associated with electronic circuits. From this starting point and the observation that the oscillation of high frequency sine waves when sustained by a small, steady supply of outside energy of the right frequency would bring about what Lakhovsky called *resonance*, he conducted experiments showing that living cells respond to oscillations imposed upon them from outside sources.

This outside source of radiation was attributed by Lakhovsky to cosmic rays that constantly bombard the earth. On the basis of these insights, Lakhovsky construed devices for healing by the application of high frequency waves, that today we know as *Radionics*.

Lakhovsky found that when outside sources of oscillations are resonating in sync with the energy code of the cell, the cell's growth would become stronger, while when frequencies differed, this would weaken the vitality of cell. From this primary observation, Lakhovsky further found that the cells of pathogenic organisms produce different frequencies than that of normal, healthy cells.

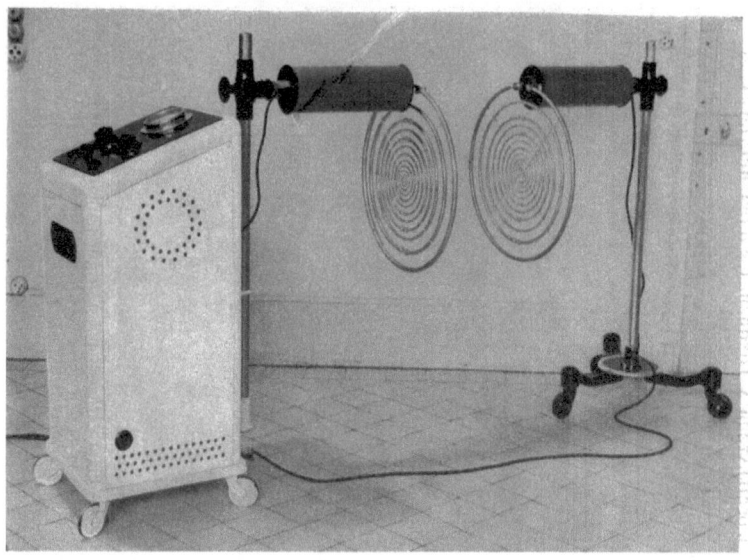

Lakhovsky specifically observed that if he could increase the amplitude, but not the frequency, of the oscillations of healthy cells, this increase would dampen the oscillations produced by disease-causing cells, thus bringing about their decline. However, when he rose the amplitude of the disease causing cells, their oscillations would gain the upper hand and cause the person or plant to become weaker and more ill. As a result of his observations, Lakhovsky viewed the progression of disease as essentially a battle between resonant oscillations of host cells versus oscillations emanating from pathogenic organisms. He initially proved his theory using plants. In December, 1924, he inoculated a set of ten germanium plants with a plant cancer that produced tumors. After thirty days, tumors had developed in all of the plants, upon which Lakhovsky took one of the ten infected plants and simply fashioned a heavy copper wire in a one loop, open-ended coil about thirty centimeter (12") in diameter around the center of the plant and held it in place. The copper coil was found to collect and concentrate energy from extremely high frequency cosmic rays.

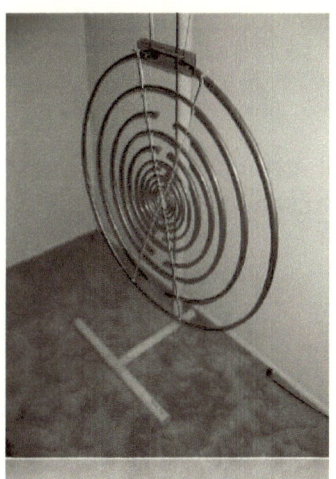

The diameter of the copper loop determined which range of frequencies would be captured. Lakhovsky found that the *thirty centimeter loop*

captured frequencies that fell within the resonant frequency range of the plant's cells.

This captured energy thus reinforced the resonant oscillations naturally produced by the nucleus of the germanium's cells. This allowed the plant to overwhelm the oscillations of the cancer cells and destroy the cancer. The tumors fell off in less than three weeks and by two months, the plant was thriving. All of the other cancer-inoculated plants, those that were not receiving the copper coil, died within thirty days.

Lakhovsky then fashioned loops of copper wire that could be worn around the waist, neck, elbows, wrists, knees, or ankles of people and found that over time relief of painful symptoms was obtained. These simple coils, worn continuously around certain parts of the body, would invigorate the vibrational strength of cells and increased the immune response which in turn took care of the offending pathogens.

Upon which Lakhovsky construed a device that produced a broad range of high frequency pulsed signals that radiate energy to the patient via two round resonators: one resonator acting as a transmitter and the other as a receiver.

RADIONICS

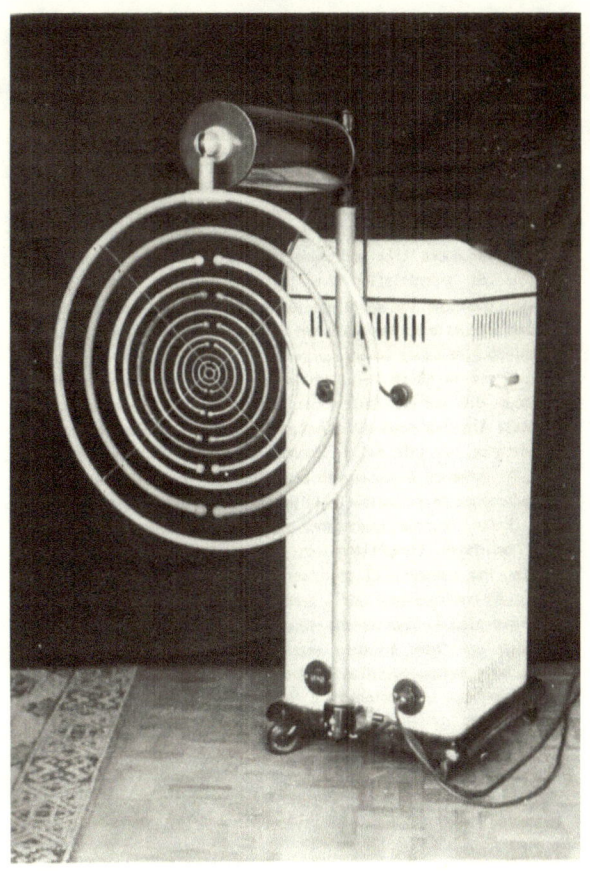

The machine generates a very wide spectrum of high frequencies coupled with static high voltage charges applied to the resonators. These high voltages cause a corona discharge around the perimeter of the outside resonator ring that Lakhovsky called *effluvia*.

The patient sat on a wooden stool in between the two resonators and was exposed to these energies for about fifteen minutes. The frequency waves *sped up the recovery process* by stimulating the resonance of healthy cells in the patient and in doing so, increased the immune response to the disease organisms.

Lakhovsky called the cosmic energy *universion*, which is the title of one of his lesser known books, published 1929 in Paris, in French language.

> —See Georges Lakhovsky, La Science et le Bonheur: Longévité et immortalité par les vibrations (1930), Le Secret de la Vie (1929), Secret of Life (2003), L'étiologie du Cancer (1929), L'Universion (1927).

Reiki

The Usui System

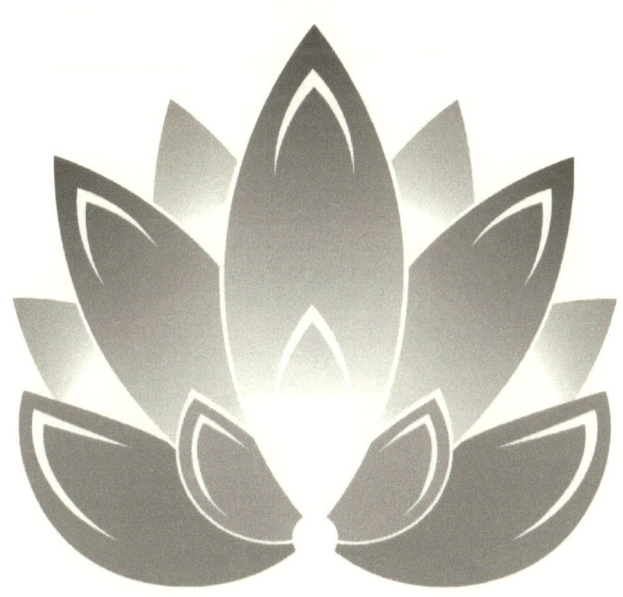

Reiki is a spiritual practice developed in 1922 by Mikao Usui. After three weeks of fasting and meditating on Mount Kurama, in Japan, Usui claimed to receive the ability of healing without energy depletion.

ALTERNATIVE MEDICINE AND WELLNESS TECHNIQUES

A portion of the practice, tenohira or palm healing, is used as a form of *complementary and alternative medicine (CAM)*. Tenohira is a technique whereby practitioners believe they are moving healing energy (a form of *ki*) through the palms.

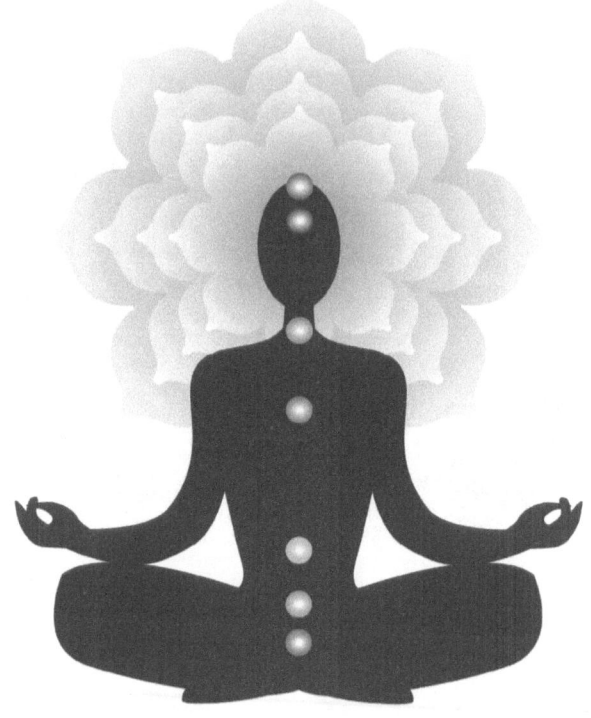

Reiki is energy-based healing. It works with what the Japanese call *ki*. Variants of energy healing exist in virtually all cultures around the world, while I must say that the Japanese have a more direct connection to it still today because of the *Shinto* religion that is one of the few in the world, next to only *Huna*, that officially recognizes psychic powers, and the invisible world, as a scientific fact, not as in dominator religions, as a religious dogma that is hammered in the minds and hearts of their believers.

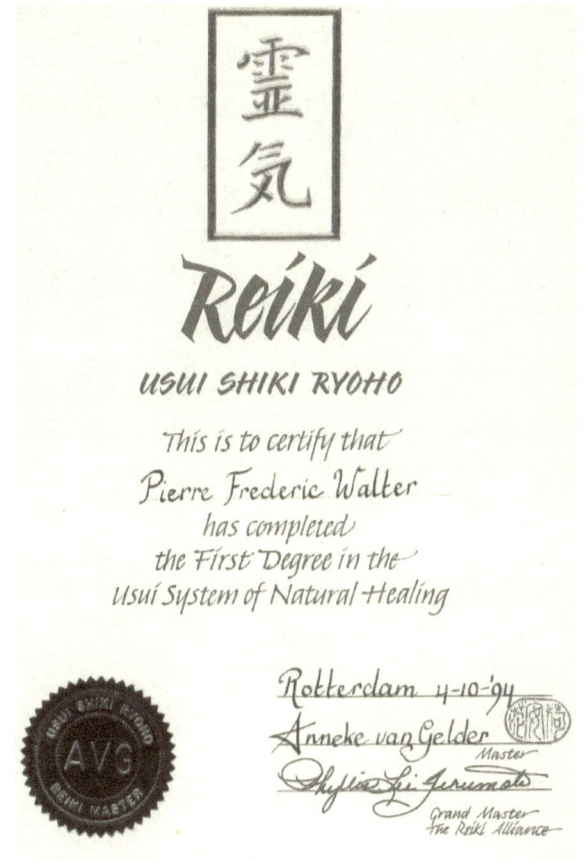

Mikao Usui has rediscovered the Reiki system at the beginning of the 20th century, while Reiki is something like a perennial natural healing technique and as such thousands of years old.

I came in touch with Reiki in 1994 through the friendship with Anneke van Gelder, a Reiki master practicing in Rotterdam, Holland, where I ran a consulting company from 1994 to 1996.

But my ideas were not really turning toward business, which is why I finally gave up that company and focused on my interests in healing and coaching people. With Anneke, then, I learnt Reiki, the whole of the theory and the practice, and to my astonishment she told me that my 'rei-ki' (from Japanese: 'intelligent energy') was very high. So I accomplished the first degree in Reiki in that year.

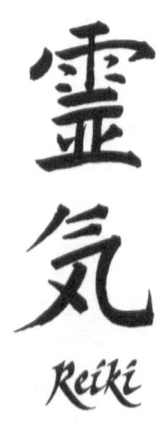

Sophrology

The Study of the Harmony of Consciousness

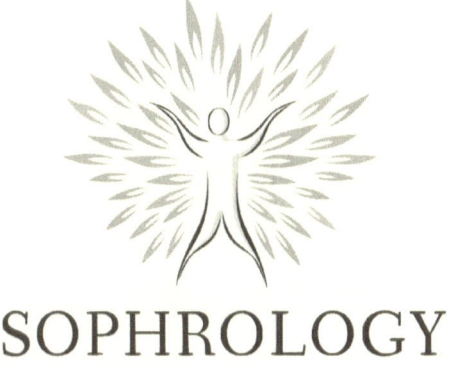

SOPHROLOGY

What is Sophrology?

Sophrology was created by Dr. Alfonso Caycedo in the 1960s. It is a branch of mindbody psychology that focuses on understanding human consciousness and altered states of consciousness for short-term or long-term positive modifications, relaxation and purposes of personal growth and creativity boosting. The term is derived from old Greek and means *study of the harmony of consciousness.*

ALTERNATIVE MEDICINE AND WELLNESS TECHNIQUES

Caycedo originally set out to find a way of healing depressed and trauma-ridden clients by leading them to health and happiness with the least possible use of drugs and psychiatric treatments. He journeyed extensively to study the Eastern philosophies of Yoga, Zen and Buddhism, each time viewing them within a Western scientific framework. Each discipline, theory and philosophy was approached with the intention of discovering what, exactly, improved people's health, both physically and mentally, in the fastest possible time and with lasting results.

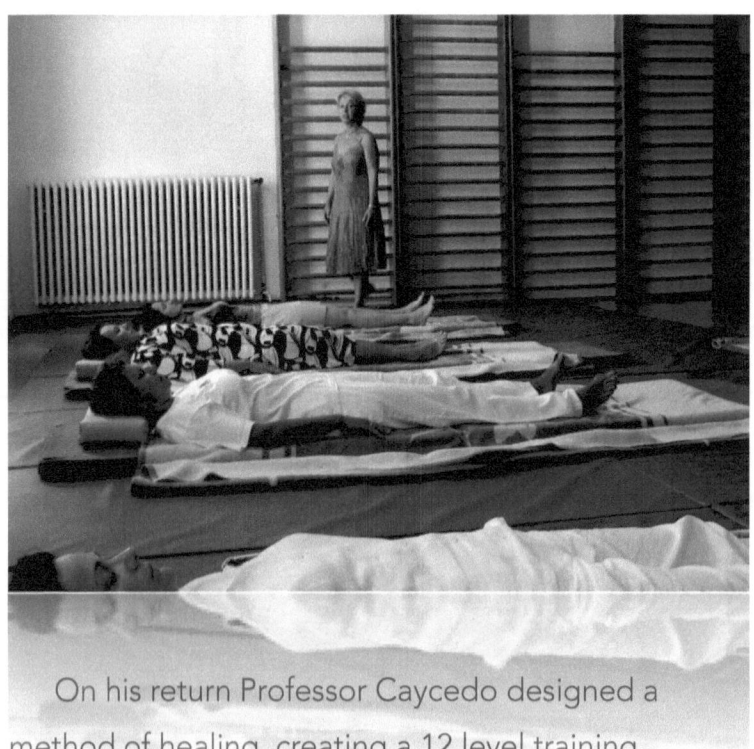

On his return Professor Caycedo designed a method of healing, creating a 12 level training program from both Eastern and Western philosophies that took into account our modern way of life—with its speed, stress and problems.

The training is divided into 3 cycles—the *reduction cycle*, the *radical cycle* and the *existential cycle*.

Professor Caycedo named his method *Sophrology* in 1960 and called it 'a training of the consciousness and the values of existence,' or 'Health & Happiness Training.'

Now, after 45 years of research, fine tuning and experimentation, he has extensive evidence of the effectiveness of the Sophrology method.

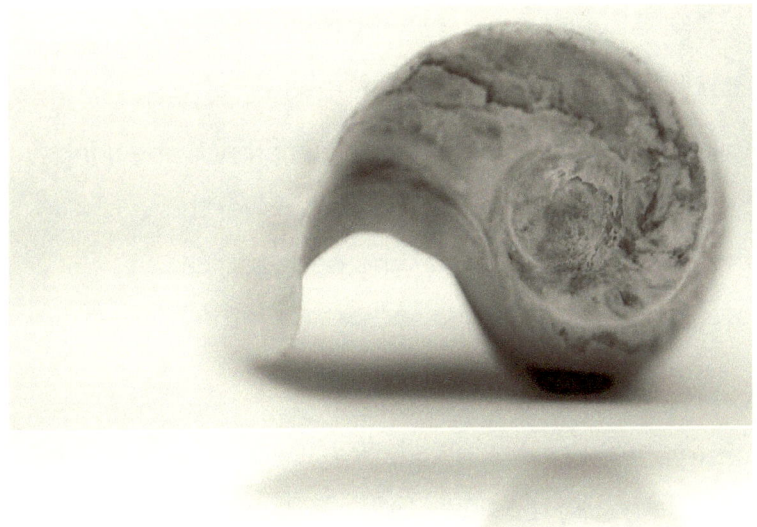

Sophrology is a structured method created to produce optimal health and wellbeing. It consists of a series of easy-to-do physical and mental exercises that, with regular practice, lead to a healthy, relaxed body and a calm, alert mind. The exercises are called *dynamic relaxation (relaxation in movement)*.

The first things people generally notice are a more restful sleep, improved concentration, fewer worries, increased self-confidence, and a feeling of inner happiness.

Statistics

Athletes coached by Dr Raymond Abrezol between 1964 and 2004 have won over 200 Olympic medals. Generally speaking, sophrology is much more common in French-speaking countries than in the Anglo-Saxon world. Here are some statistics that show it.

Over 300,000 members of the public have followed courses of sophrology in French-speaking Switzerland over the last 25 years. Over three thousand medical, social and pedagogical professionals have followed the train-the-trainers lessons.

Sophrology was initially firmly within the field of psychiatry and medicine until Dr Raymond Abrezol discovered its unique benefits, and brought it to the attention of the great public.

After practicing Sophrology for a while, Dr Abrezol began to observe a noticeable improvement in his tennis game. As an experiment, he introduced his opponents to the method, and they began to see their tennis vastly improve. He was consequently invited to coach the Swiss ski team and other Olympic athletes.

The rapid growth of Sophrology throughout the French-speaking world can largely be attributed to Dr Abrezol running trainer training programs for a large number of influential doctors and sports coaches, many of whom now run centers throughout France. His enthusiasm and his success with athletes opened doors for Sophrology to be taught in many areas of life.

Benefits

Sophrology assists to rediscover our self-confidence and hidden potential. Group classes bring improvements in communications and interpersonal relations.

Students have a stronger resistance to stressful situations, whether mental or physical. Since they have many more choices of how to act and react, it is easier to break out of old habitual patterns into more successful ways of operating.

The most important part is regular practice until the benefits of the Sophrology Training become part of everyday life.

Tai Chi Chuan

The Soft Martial Art

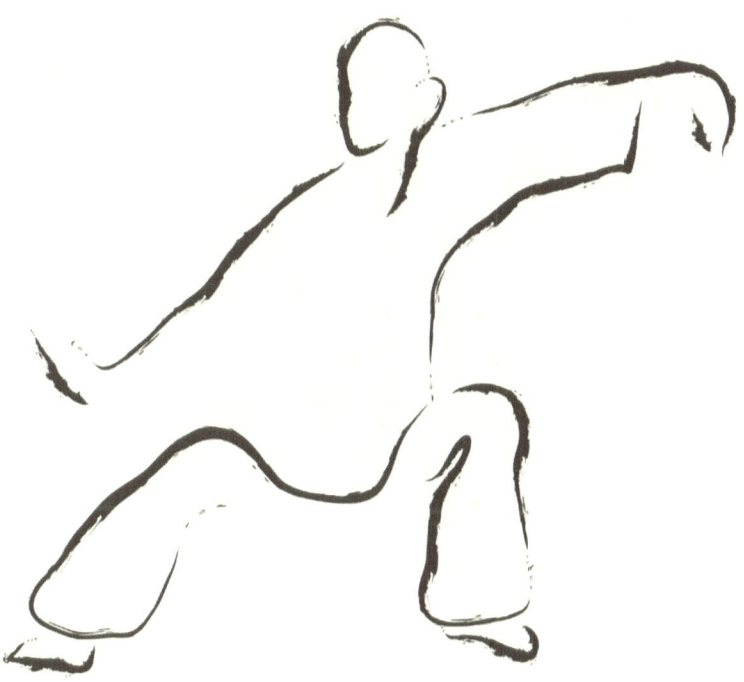

What is Tai Chi Chuan?

Tai Chi Chuan is an internal Chinese martial art, often promoted and practiced as a martial arts therapy for the purposes of health and longevity.

ALTERNATIVE MEDICINE AND WELLNESS TECHNIQUES

Tai Chi Chuan is considered a soft style martial art, an art applied with as much deep relaxation or softness in the musculature as possible, to distinguish its theory and application from that of the hard martial art styles which use a degree of tension in the muscles. Variations of basic training forms are well known as the slow motion routines that groups of people practice every morning in parks across China and other parts of the world.

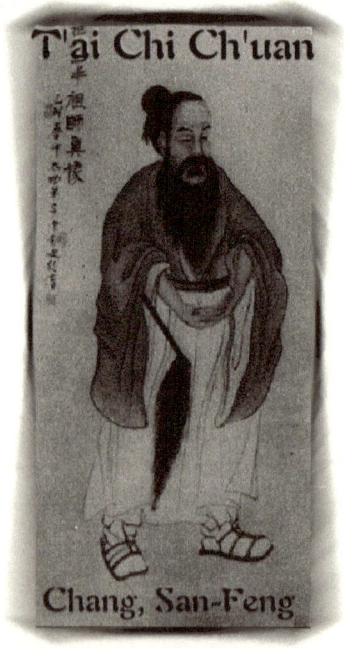

TAI CHI CHUAN

Traditional Tai Chi training is intended to teach awareness of one's energy balance and what affects it, awareness of the same in others, an appreciation of the practical value in one's ability to moderate extremes of behavior and attitude at both mental and physical levels, and how this applies to effective self-defense principles.

Based on softness and awareness, rather than force and resistance, Tai Chi Chuan has been recognized for thousands of years as both a method of self-cultivation and an unexcelled form of self-defense.

The Movements

Tai Chi Chuan is a noncompetitive, self-paced system of gentle physical exercise and stretching. You perform a series of postures or movements in a slow, graceful manner.

Each posture flows into the next without pausing.

Anyone, regardless of age or physical ability, can practice these movements as they require awareness rather than strength, and they can be done effortlessly. It doesn't take physical prowess.

The Benefits

—Reduce stress

—Increase flexibility

—Improve muscle strength and definition

—Increase energy, stamina and agility

—Increase your general sense of wellbeing

Tai Chi Chuan knows more than one hundred possible movements and positions. You can find several that you like, and stick with those, or explore the full range.

The intensity of the movements varies somewhat depending on the form or style practiced. Some forms are more fast-paced than others, for instance. However, most forms are gentle and suitable for everyone. And they all include *rhythmic patterns of movement* that are to be coordinated with breathing.

TAI CHI CHUAN

Like other practices that bring mind and body together, the practice of Tai Chi Chuan reduces stress.

When you do the movements, you focus on movement and breathing. This combination creates a state of relaxation and calm. Stress, anxiety and tension should melt away as you focus on the present, and the effects may last well after you stop your session.

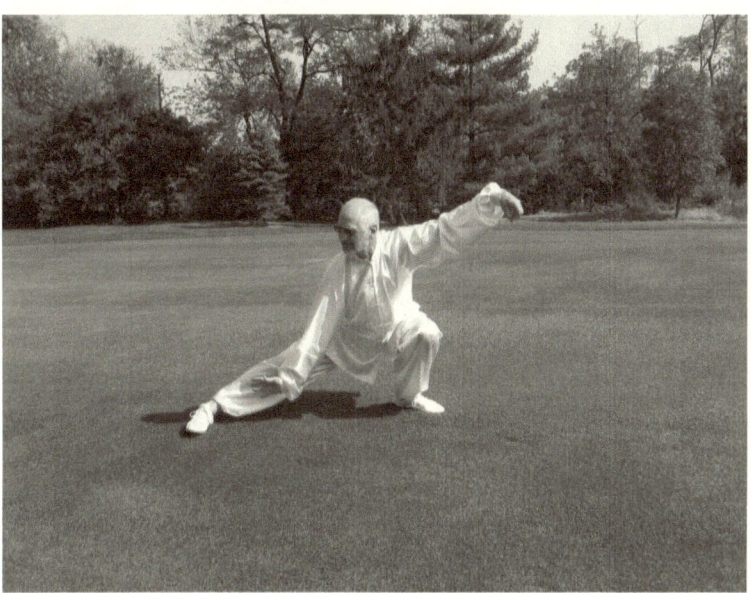

Tai Chi Chuan may also help your overall health, although it's not a substitute for traditional medical care, but rather a form of prophylaxis.

Tai Chi Chuan is generally safe for people of all ages and levels of fitness. Older adults may especially find it appealing because the movements are low impact and put minimal stress on muscles and joints.

Tai Chi Chuan may also be helpful if you have arthritis or are recovering from an injury.

Learning the Technique

Wondering how to get started? You don't need any special clothing or equipment. To gain full benefits, however, it may be best to seek guidance from a qualified instructor, who can teach you specific positions and how to regulate your breathing.

An instructor also can teach you how to practice safely, especially if you have injuries, chronic conditions, or balance or coordination problems.

Practice Regularly

To reap the greatest stress reduction benefits from Tai Chi Chuan, consider practicing it regularly.

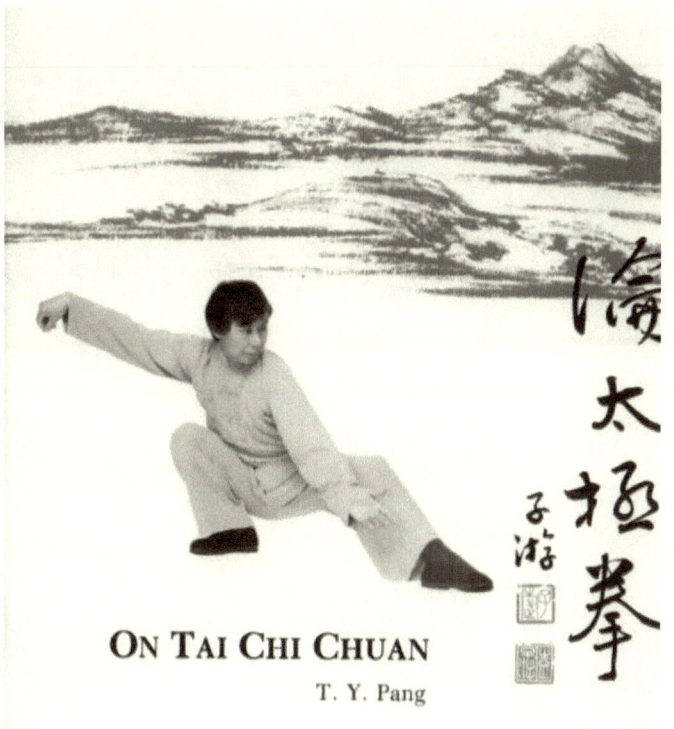

Many people find it helpful to practice in the same place and at the same time every day to develop a routine. But if your schedule is erratic, do your cycle whenever you have a few minutes.

You can even draw on the soothing concepts of Tai Chi Chuan without performing the actual movements if you get stuck in stressful situations—a traffic jam or a work conflict, for instance. You can do your movements in your mind, for example, remembering the feelings of wellbeing that you experienced when doing it last time.

The Tai Chi Chuan movements are widely acknowledged to help calm the emotions, focus the mind, and strengthen the immune system. In a very real sense, it helps us to stay younger as we grow older, thus making an outstanding contribution to our overall health and wellbeing.

Meaning of the Word

The term *Tai Chi Chuan* literally translates as 'supreme ultimate fist,' 'boundless fist,' 'great extremes boxing,' or simply 'the ultimate.'

Tai Chi Chuan is generally classified as a form of traditional Chinese martial arts of the soft or internal branch. It is considered a soft style martial art, an art applied with internal power, to distinguish its theory and application from that of the hard martial art styles.

Tai Chi Chuan, by Master Shou-Yu Liang

This is a review of Master Liang's outstanding book and DVD entitled *Tai Chi Chuan, 24 & 48 Postures with*

TAI CHI CHUAN

Martial Applications, Roslindale: YMAA Publication Center, 1996.

Before I purchased book and DVD on amazon.com, I was reading to of the reviews, and publish them here, as I find them well-written and to the point:

Midwest Book Review
One of China's top-ranked coaches to Tai Chi provides an illustrated guide to the 24 and 48 postures, including tips on breathing, aligning the body, and developing Chi. Martial applications are also surveyed in a presentation notable for its many step-by-step black and white photos which excel in illustrating positions and movements.

Duane
The simplified, widely practiced 24-posture form was devised by the Chinese government in the 1950's due to a shortage of doctors. Founded primarily on the Yang style, it takes 5–10 minutes to practice, less time than for the 37- and 108-posture forms.

Yang style is probably the most thoroughly documented style of Taijiquan, for better or worse. So this 24-posture short version represents a mainstream starting point.

Liang's compact manual probably offers the most complete and concise description of this form available, together with overview of historical background, training tips, and illustrations of martial applications "hidden" within the form.

The companion video of the same name (purchased separately) shows the sequence twice from the front view, once from the back. Then it shows martial applications individually and also the 48-posture version. To get the 24-posture form broken down in detail, I also recommend Dr. Paul Lam's DVD, 'Tai Chi the 24 forms.'

In the YMAA tradition of Dr. Yang, this manual (and video) represent training notes at a disciplined, somewhat demanding level. The numbering system for the photographs, together with the compactness of the page layout have caused me to pencil in some arrows and titles. If you're simply looking for a group stretching routine to follow along with at your local community center, you may consider this text ambitious.

It was the above-quoted book review by Mr. C. Duane, that is published on amazon.com that gave the trigger to my buying this book, and the corresponding DVD.

I was positively surprised when I received the book and DVD.

What I found especially useful are the black arrows that trace all the movements to be made.

In addition, you see them performed by Master Liang on the DVD, and further, there is a meticulous description simultaneous to the movements, in English, to be heard on the DVD.

I can't imagine how to do it better; this is simply the best form of pedagogy for learning Tai Chi—which is if you want to do it in the right way, not in the Western way, *not easy* to learn. It requires full attention to detail and a fully developed body consciousness. And that is exactly what it develops in the first place. It raises our body consciousness or what I came to term *emonic consciousness*, because it implies awareness of the *ch'i*, the vital energy flow in the organism. The author introduces the book with the following elucidation that I think is worth to be quoted:

'Chinese view the universe as one interrelated organism, not as separate entities; everything resonates with each other to reach balance and harmony. This view, on a smaller scale, also applies to the human body. It is believed that studying the universe will give us an understanding of the small universe—the human body. /2'

Indeed, what our new science is now discovering was known to the Chinese already more than five thousand years ago. So there is nothing new under the sun, in fact. The only difference between ancient China and our times in this context is the fact that they called knowledge 'philosophy,' while we today call it 'science,' but these expressions actually mean the same.

And the parallel goes even farther. The ancient Chinese sages knew that knowledge alone, as long as it's mere theory or concepts, will not really foster human evolution; what is further needed is to align our breath with the cosmic breath, and this was done, in China, through Qigong, and Tai Chi Chuan.

ALTERNATIVE MEDICINE AND WELLNESS TECHNIQUES

All Eastern martial arts are in essence breathing exercises; all movements are done with the ultimate purpose of teaching us how to breathe properly.

And in the West, many managers and high-grade officials have discovered in a process that goes over the last two or three decades that knowledge and skills alone will not make a really powerful, effective, human, and wistful manager. And that is why, naturally, managers and leaders from all walks of life nowadays discover *mindbody coordinating techniques,* such as Zen, Qigong and Tai Chi Chuan, and some others.

There is a fast growing awareness since the 1990s that these techniques actually are a must for whoever is in a position of leading others, for moral integrity is one of the finest elements of these techniques since the oldest traditions, as it was known since the beginnings of human history that a good leader can only be one who has achieved moral integrity at a high and even outstanding level.

What is this moral integrity about? Beware, it is not what I came to call *moralism,* and it is not judging others and life, it is not persecuting others because they have different sexual tastes, and it is not splitting life in a good-and-bad scheme. It is *true* morality, not the fake many Westerners are addicted to and that they call 'good behavior' or 'decency.'

It is nothing of all that. It is integrity, and acceptance; it is intelligent and nonjudgmental understanding at a very high level. It is also compassion, empathy with self and others, tolerance, and emotional maturity.

Master Liang says that training the mind is of the highest importance for the practice of Tai Chi Chuan. And this is naturally so because what happens when we train the mind is that we *build awareness of our projections* that grow out from our blind spots and moral weaknesses. Master Liang formulates moral integrity in these rather pragmatic terms:

> To achieve the maximum benefit from Taijiquan practice, you should 'practice Taijiquan 24 hours a day.' This doesn't mean that you need to do the Taijiquan sequence all the time, but you need to make Taijiquan a way of life. The practice of Taijiquan will not only provide a 'whole' body workout; but also cultivate the energy within your body, increase your mental awareness and centering, and build good habits for proper body alignment. When you have accomplished these goals in practice, you will automatically carry these good habits into your daily life. You will gain a greater awareness of yourself; keeping your physical

body properly aligned while sitting, standing, driving, eating, watching TV, working, typing, brushing your teeth, and everything else you do regularly. This is what is meant by 'practicing Taijiquan 24 hours a day' and 'making Taijiquan a way of life.'/15

Tibetan Medicine

Feeling the Pulse

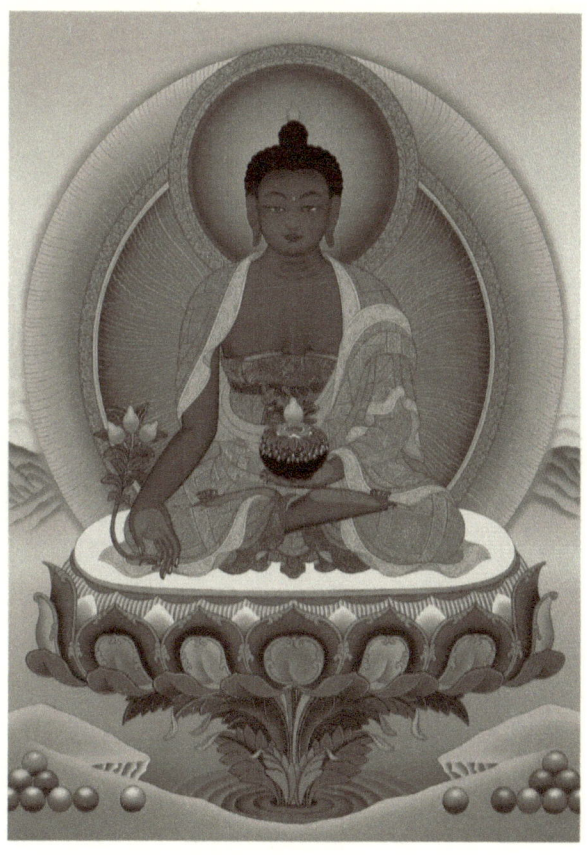

I discovered Tibetan traditional medicine in 1994, in the Netherlands. I had suffered from a long-lasting pain in my right knee that no Western doctor could heal, and my Chinese friends in Rotterdam sent me to a Tibetan healer in Amsterdam.

While all the Western doctors had diagnosed some or the other local problem with the ligaments, the Tibetan healer, after feeling my pulse for quite a long moment, said there was nothing wrong with my knee's ligaments, and the problem was instead a *cold spot* that probably was caused through uncovering myself during sleep.

I was rather suspicious to this diagnosis as it sounded so simplistic, but followed the advice of the healer to wear a *simple woolen bandage* around the knee for a minimum of two weeks.

In addition, he gave me a herbal balm that was, as he said, keeping my knee warm, and advised me to once in a while take a warm bath. To my surprise, after two or three weeks, the pain was gone and was never any more coming up thereafter.

And the doctor, despite my insisting upon paying his fee, refused to accept any payment, despite the fact that in addition to one hour of consultation, he had given me the balm and the woolen bandage for free.

TIBETAN MEDICINE

As I had been recommended by friends, he explained, he was not supposed to accept any payment. I did not need further elucidation about the *professional ethics*, the competence and the supreme level of virtue of Tibetan natural healers.

Yoga

The Two Yoga

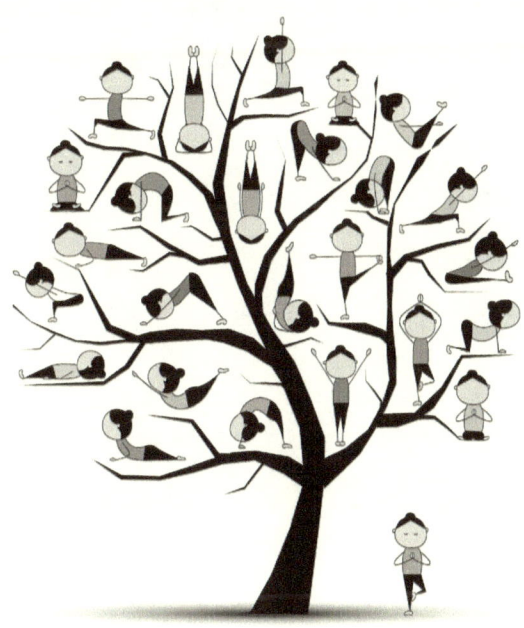

Indian Yoga

The word Yoga means to join or unite. It is generally translated as union of the individual *atman* or individual soul with *paramatman* or *brahman* or universal soul.

Yoga is a family of ancient spiritual practices dating back more than five thousand years from India. It is one of the six schools of Hindu philosophy. In India, Yoga is seen as a means to both physiological and spiritual mastery. Outside of India, Yoga has become primarily associated with the practice of *asanas (postures)* of Hatha Yoga.

Yoga as a means of spiritual attainment is central to Hinduism, Buddhism and Jainism and has influenced other religious and spiritual practices throughout the world. Hindu texts establishing the basis for yoga include the *Upanishads*, the *Bhagavad Gita*, the *Yoga Sutras of Patanjali*, the *Hatha Yoga Pradipika* and many others.

The four main paths of Yoga are *Karma Yoga, Jnana Yoga, Bhakti Yoga* and *Raja Yoga*. Practitioners of yoga are referred to as a *yogi* or *yogin* (male), and *yogini* (female).

CHINESE-THAI YOGA

Tao Yoga is a method coined by the Thai-American Master Mantak Chia that consists in directing the bioenergetic flow of the organism by means of mental focus and deep breathing. Mantak Chia has explained and illustrated the method and its application extensively in his books.

BIBLIOGRAPHY

Contextual Bibliography

ARNTZ, WILLIAM & CHASSE, BETSY

What the Bleep Do We Know
20th Century Fox, 2005 (DVD)

Down The Rabbit Hole Quantum Edition
20th Century Fox, 2006 (3 DVD Set)

BERTALANFFY, LUDWIG VON

General Systems Theory
Foundations, Development, Applications
New York: George Brazilier Publishing, 1976

BORDEAUX-SZEKELY, EDMOND

Teaching of the Essenes from Enoch to the Dead
Sea Scrolls
Beekman Publishing, 1992

Gospel of the Essenes
The Unknown Books of the Essenes & Lost Scrolls of the Essene Brotherhood
Beekman Publishing, 1988

Gospel of Peace of Jesus Christ
Beekman Publishing, 1994

Gospel of Peace, 2d Vol.
I B S International Publishers

ALTERNATIVE MEDICINE AND WELLNESS TECHNIQUES

Brennan, Barbara Ann

Hands of Healing
A Guide to Healing Through the Human Energy Field
New York: Bantam, 1988

Capra, Bernt Amadeus

Mindwalk
A Film for Passionate Thinkers
Based Upon Fritjof Capra's *The Turning Point*
New York: Triton Pictures, 1990

Capra, Fritjof

The Turning Point
Science, Society And The Rising Culture
New York: Simon & Schuster, 1987
Original Author Copyright, 1982

The Tao of Physics
An Exploration of the Parallels Between Modern
Physics and Eastern Mysticism
New York: Shambhala Publications, 2000
(New Edition) Originally published in 1975

The Web of Life
A New Scientific Understanding of Living Systems
New York: Doubleday, 1997

The Hidden Connections
Integrating The Biological, Cognitive And Social
Dimensions Of Life Into A Science Of Sustainability
New York: Doubleday, 2002

CONTEXTUAL BIBLIOGRAPHY

Steering Business Toward Sustainability
New York: United Nations University Press, 1995

Uncommon Wisdom
Conversations with Remarkable People
New York: Bantam, 1989

The Science of Leonardo
Inside the Mind of the Great Genius of the Renaissance
New York: Anchor Books, 2008
New York: Bantam Doubleday, 2007 (First Publishing)

CHIA, MANTAK

Taoist Ways to Transform Stress into Vitality
Chi Self-Massage
Huntington: The Healing Tao Press, 1985

Awaken Healing Energy through the Tao
The Taoist Secret of Circulating Internal Power
New York: Aurora Press, 1983

CRAZE, RICHARD

Feng Shui
Feng Shui Book & Card Pack
London: Thorsons, 1997

EDEN, DONNA & FEINSTEIN, DAVID

Energy Medicine
New York: Tarcher/Putnam, 1998

The Energy Medicine Kit
Simple Effective Techniques to Help You Boost Your Vitality

ALTERNATIVE MEDICINE AND WELLNESS TECHNIQUES

Boulder, Co.: Sounds True Editions, 2004

The Promise of Energy Psychology
With David Feinstein and Gary Craig
Revolutionary Tools for Dramatic Personal Change
New York: Jeremy P. Tarcher/Penguin, 2005

EMOTO, MASARU

The Hidden Messages in Water
New York: Atria Books, 2004

The Secret Life of Water
New York: Atria Books, 2005

GERBER, RICHARD

A Practical Guide to Vibrational Medicine
Energy Healing and Spiritual Transformation
New York: Harper & Collins, 2001

HALL, MANLY P.

The Pineal Gland
The Eye of God
Kessinger Publishing Reprint

The Secret Teachings of All Ages
Reader's Edition
New York: Tarcher/Penguin, 2003
Originally published in 1928

CONTEXTUAL BIBLIOGRAPHY

Goswami, Amit

The Self-Aware Universe
How Consciousness Creates the Material World
New York: Tarcher/Putnam, 1995

Herrigel, Eugen

Zen in the Art of Archery
New York: Vintage Books, 1999
Originally published in 1971

Hunt, Valerie

Infinite Mind
Science of the Human Vibrations of Consciousness
Malibu, CA: Malibu Publishing, 2000

Huxley, Aldous

The Doors of Perception and Heaven and Hell
London: HarperCollins (Flamingo), 1994
(originally published in 1954)

The Perennial Philosophy
San Francisco: Harper & Row, 1970

Kapleau, Roshi Philip

Three Pillars of Zen
Boston: Beacon Press, 1967

ALTERNATIVE MEDICINE AND WELLNESS TECHNIQUES

Karagulla, Shafica

The Chakras
Correlations between Medical Science and Clairvoyant Observation
With Dora van Gelder Kunz
Wheaton: Quest Books, 1989

Kerner, Justinus

F.A. Mesmer aus Schwaben
Frankfurt/M, 1856

Kiesewetter, Carl

Franz Anton Mesmer's Leben und Lehre
Leipzig, 1893

Kingston, Karen

Creating Sacred Space With Feng Shui
New York: Broadway Books, 1997

Kwok, Man-Ho

The Feng Shui Kit
London: Piatkus, 1995

Lakhovsky, Georges

La Science et le Bonheur
Longévité et Immortalité par les Vibrations
Paris: Gauthier-Villars, 1930

CONTEXTUAL BIBLIOGRAPHY

Le Secret de la Vie
Paris: Gauthier-Villars, 1929

Secret of Life
New York: Kessinger Publishing, 2003
First published in 1929

L'étiologie du Cancer
Paris: Gauthier-Villars, 1929

L'Universion
Paris: Gauthier-Villars, 1927

LASZLO, ERVIN

Science and the Akashic Field
An Integral Theory of Everything
Rochester: Inner Traditions, 2004

Quantum Shift to the Global Brain
How the New Scientific Reality Can Change Us and Our World
Rochester: Inner Traditions, 2008

Science and the Reenchantment of the Cosmos
The Rise of the Integral Vision of Reality
Rochester: Inner Traditions, 2006

The Akashic Experience
Science and the Cosmic Memory Field
Rochester: Inner Traditions, 2009

The Chaos Point
The World at the Crossroads
Newburyport, MA: Hampton Roads Publishing, 2006

ALTERNATIVE MEDICINE AND WELLNESS TECHNIQUES

Liedloff, Jean

Continuum Concept
In Search of Happiness Lost
New York: Perseus Books, 1986
First published in 1977

Long, Max Freedom

The Secret Science at Work
The Huna Method as a Way of Life
Marina del Rey: De Vorss Publications, 1995
Originally published in 1953

Growing Into Light
A Personal Guide to Practicing the Huna Method,
Marina del Rey: De Vorss Publications, 1955

Master Lam Kam Chuen

The Way of Energy
Mastering the Chinese Art of Internal
Strength with Chi Kung Exercise
New York: Simon & Schuster (Fireside), 1991

Master Liang, Shou-Yu & Wu, Wen-Ching

Tai Chi Chuan
24 & 48 Postures With Martial Applications
Roslindale, Mass.: YMAA Publication Center, 1996

CONTEXTUAL BIBLIOGRAPHY

McCarey, William A.

In Search of Healing
Whole-Body Healing Through the Mind-Body-Spirit Connection
New York: Berkley Publishing, 1996

McTaggart, Lynne

The Field
The Quest for the Secret Force of the Universe
New York: Harper & Collins, 2002

Meadows, Donella H.

Thinking in Systems
A Primer
White River, VT: Chelsea Green Publishing, 2008

Myss, Caroline

The Creation of Health
The Emotional, Psychological, and Spiritual Responses that Promote Health and Healing
New York: Three Rivers Press, 1998

Nau, Erika

Self-Awareness Through Huna
Virginia Beach: Donning, 1981

ALTERNATIVE MEDICINE AND WELLNESS TECHNIQUES

Ni, Hua-Ching

I Ching

The Book of Changes and the Unchanging Truth
2nd edition
Santa Barbara: Seven Star Communications, 1999

Esoteric Tao The Ching
The Shrine of the Eternal Breath of Tao
Santa Monica: College of Tao and Traditional Chinese Healing, 1992

The Complete Works of Lao Tzu
Tao The Ching & Hua Hu Ching
Translation and Elucidation by Hua-Ching Ni
Santa Monica: Seven Star Communications, 1995

Ni, Maoshing

The Tao of Nutrition
3rd Edition
With Cathy McNease
Los Angeles: Tao of Wellness, 2012

Ong, Hean-Tatt

Amazing Scientific Basis of Feng Shui
Kuala Lumpur: Eastern Dragon Press, 1997

Ponder, Catherine

The Healing Secrets of the Ages
Marine del Rey: DeVorss, 1985

CONTEXTUAL BIBLIOGRAPHY

REID, DANIEL P.

The Tao of Health, Sex & Longevity
A Modern Practical Guide to the Ancient Way
New York: Simon & Schuster, 1989

Guarding the Three Treasures
The Chinese Way of Health
New York: Simon & Schuster, 1993

SANTOPIETRO, NANCY

Feng Shui, Harmony by Design
How to Create a Beautiful and Harmonious Home
New York: Putnam-Berkeley, 1996

SCHULTES, RICHARD EVANS, ET AL.

Plants of the Gods
Their Sacred, Healing, and Hallucinogenic Powers
New York: Healing Arts Press
2nd edition, 2002

SHELDRAKE, RUPERT

A New Science of Life
The Hypothesis of Morphic Resonance
Rochester: Park Street Press, 1995

SIMONTON, O. CARL ET AL.

Getting Well Again
Los Angeles: Tarcher, 1978

STIENE, BRONWEN & FRANS

The Reiki Sourcebook
New York: O Books, 2003

The Japanese Art of Reiki
A Practical Guide to Self-Healing
New York: O Books, 2005

TALBOT, MICHAEL

The Holographic Universe
New York: HarperCollins, 1992

TANSLEY, DAVID V.

Chakras, Rays and Radionics
London: Daniel Company Ltd., 1984

TATAR, MARIA M.

Spellbound: Studies on Mesmerism and Literature
Princeton, N.Y., 1978

TILLER, WILLIAM A.

Conscious Acts of Creation
The Emergence of a New Physics
Associated Producers, 2004 (DVD)

Psychoenergetic Science
New York: Pavior, 2007

Conscious Acts of Creation
New York: Pavior, 2001

CONTEXTUAL BIBLIOGRAPHY

Too, Lillian

Feng Shui
Kuala Lumpur: Konsep Books, 1994

Walker, N.W.

The Natural Way to Vibrant Health
Prescott, AZ: Norwalk Press, 1972

Watson, George

Nutrition and Your Mind
The Psychochemical Response
New York: Harper & Row, 1972

Watts, Alan W.

The Way of Zen
New York: Vintage Books, 1999

This Is It
And Other Essays on Zen and Spiritual Experience
New York: Vintage, 1973

Wydra, Nancilee

Feng Shui
The Book of Cures
Lincolnwood: Contemporary Books, 1996

ALTERNATIVE MEDICINE AND WELLNESS TECHNIQUES

Yang, Jwing-Ming

Qigong, The Secret of Youth
Da Mo's Muscle/Tendon Changing and Marrow/Brain Washing Classics
Boston, Mass.: YMAA Publication Center, 2000

The Root of Chinese Qigong
Secrets for Health, Longevity, & Enlightenment
Roslindale, MA: YMAA Publication Center, 1997

Young, Robert O.

The pH Miracle
Balance Your Diet, Reclaim Your Health
With Shelley Redford Young
New York: Grand Central Life & Style, 2010

Personal Notes

www.ingramcontent.com/pod-product-compliance
Lightning Source LLC
Chambersburg PA
CBHW031051180526
45163CB00002BA/783